Medicine & Society
In America

*Medicine & Society
In America*

Advisory Editor

Charles E. Rosenberg
Professor of History
University of Pennsylvania

THE

PHYSIOLOGY OF MARRIAGE.

BY
WILLIAM A. ALCOTT, M.D.,

Introduction by
Charles E. Rosenberg

*A*RNO *P*RESS & *T*HE *N*EW *Y*ORK *T*IMES
New York 1972

Reprint Edition 1972 by Arno Press Inc.

Introduction Copyright © 1972 by
Charles E. Rosenberg

Reprinted from a copy in
The Library of The College of
Physicians of Philadelphia

LC# 79-180551
ISBN 0-405-03931-X

Medicine and Society in America
ISBN for complete set: 0-405-03930-1
See last pages of this volume for titles.

Manufactured in the United States of America

INTRODUCTION

Dr. William Alcott is almost unknown today, though his cousin Bronson and Bronson's daughter Louisa May Alcott are familiar names to students of American culture. Yet in the generation before the Civil War, William Alcott was one of America's most widely read authors—not of fiction, but of popular health and educational guides. Indefatigable, he turned out fifty books on hygiene and education for adults, plus almost as many more for children. Whether aimed at the "young mother," "young husband," "young man," or "young wife," Alcott's little treatises always incorporated a characteristically Jacksonian mixture of pious and materialistic reform, an uncompromising and almost ingenuous faith in man's ability to understand, control, and improve his life. Vegetarianism, phrenology, and a prudent regimen generally were means to a holier, a healthier, and ultimately even a perfect life.

Within this tradition of concern for health and moral improvement, Alcott's *Physiology of Marriage* is perhaps his most important and revealing book,* for it not only illustrates the nature of Alcott's reformist commitment but demonstrates as well the deeply ambivalent concern of middle-class Americans with the physical aspect of marriage. *The Physiology of Marriage* is, in other words, a "sex manual," a guide to the perplexed in an area peculiarly defined by anxiety and perplexity.

Despite the traditional cliche that Victorians never discussed—and barely practiced—the physical aspects of sex, Alcott's book makes clear the prominent role played by sexuality in contemporary social reality. He was well aware of the nature and variety of American sexual behavior, including not only widespread prostitution and abortion, but even sodomy. (Alcott could not be sure of the prevalence of the latter in heterosexual relationships but was well aware of its existence in prisons.) On the other hand, Alcott's evangelical suspicion of sexuality does represent a genuine and pervasive reality in mid-nineteenth-century America. Though Alcott knew well enough that sex was probably the most anxiety-provoking concern in the minds

*The first edition was published anonymously; later editions bore Alcott's name.

of young people contemplating marriage, he sought to temper their natural "ardency" and explain the dangers of imprudent and excessive utilization of the sexual powers—within as well as outside marriage. Thus, one of the more elaborate discussions in the *Physiology of Marriage* concerns the appropriate frequency for sexual intercourse. In endorsing "once a month" as a realistic expectation, Alcott actually steered a middle course within the evangelical camp. John Cowan, a somewhat more millennial enthusiast, suggested instead that sexual intercourse be indulged in only when children were actually desired and conception was possible. With pregnancy, lactation, and an appropriate period of recuperation for the mother, the intervals between sexual indulgence, he declared, might be as long as three years.

Birth control and abortion were other realities of mid-nineteenth-century marriage. Here Alcott also assumed a moderate stance. Though unqualifiedly opposing abortion and mechanical means of birth control, he does concede that the prudent spacing of children might well be necessary, that abstinence was in most cases an unrealistic goal, and that either the rhythm method or withdrawal constituted acceptable compromises. Many of his contemporaries (especially those writing in the years after 1870) found reasons to oppose withdrawal, which some termed "conjugal onanism," and indeed all modes of birth control as not only immoral but physically debilitating.

In rejecting the plausibility of abstinence as a means of birth control, Alcott was simply expressing the popular assumption that sexual activity was a normal, if not indeed a necessary, part of human physiology. The existence of a function implied use; certainly this was the case with men. With regard to women, however, Alcott displayed an ambivalence characteristic of his generation. Though he denied formally that normal women ordinarily felt sexual desire, his discussions of actual behavior indicate Alcott's casual awareness that women did indeed feel such desire. Even in women past the childbearing age, he noted, for example, that sexual desire persisted. In a passage proscribing sexual intercourse during pregnancy, Alcott warned that it was somewhat injurious to the fetus, but that if the mother experienced pleasure it was far more dangerous: "The nervous orgasm is too much for the young germ." (Such ideological formulations make the temptation to indulge in psycho-history almost overpowering. The male child's Oedipal anxieties and fear of female sexuality would appear to be thus neatly expressed in Alcott's intellectual ideogram—the mother dramatically betraying the child within her in succumbing to the father's sexual desire.)

The need for control was clearly a dominant motif in Alcott's view of sexuality. And perhaps this emphasis was implied by the structural realities of mid-nineteenth-century life. The need for late marriage and the danger of premature and excessive childbearing in a society in which economic life was highly labile and social status was chronically insecure made self-control in sexual matters (as in economic matters) a necessity. Hence the stern and universal warnings in Alcott's generation against sexual activity during adolescence, and the prevalence of similar warnings against the turning of the marriage bed into a field for the unbridled exercise of sexual desire. Thus, possibly, the seemingly compulsive and stylized warnings against masturbation in both sexes (what could more clearly embody loss of control and a surrender to private, antisocial indulgence). Historians have become increasingly aware of the significant emotional nexus between economic and sexual images in the rhetoric of mid-nineteenth-century physicians and social commentators concerned with sexual matters.

In some ways as interesting as Alcott's injunctions are the sanctions he employs in enforcing them. He almost never resorts to categorical spiritual arguments. God does not strike the fornicator, masturbator, or married sybarite directly; nor are his punishments limited to the sphere of the eternal. It is the lecher's own abuse of his God-given capacities that brings inevitable punishment. Thus, in his warnings against "marital excess," Alcott employs thoroughly pragmatic—if not indeed cynical —arguments. He promises, for example, that prudent intervals between sexual intercourse would result in greater physical pleasure when it was performed, and that postponement of sexual activity in youth would result in an extended capacity to feel pleasure in one's middle and old age.

Alcott explained again and again that there could be no inconsistency between the material laws of man's being and God's eternal commandments. This argument was, of course, traditional; but Alcott's particular emphasis on the sufficiency of bodily salvation is rather peculiar. It is by no means a simple secularism, for Alcott's secular goals are always suffused with a transcendent justification. Thus, when discussing the hereditary consequences of right living (or its lack), Alcott asked rhetorically:

> Whose heart does not beat high at the bare possibility of becoming the progenitor of a world,

> as it were, of pure, holy, healthy, and greatly elevated beings—a race worthy of emerging from the fall—and of enstamping on it a species of immortality?

Obedience to physiological laws would ultimately create a race of men capable of cooperating with the Son of God in the redemption of the human race in "body, soul, and spirit."

Alcott's habitual use of hereditary sanctions in enforcing the dictates of morality was particularly novel—and characteristic of arguments to become increasingly popular in the second half of the nineteenth century. Thus the thoughtful care of women during pregnancy (of course, eschewing intercourse) was urged as a necessity if healthy and moral offspring were to be produced. Similarly, sexual activity during the early part of lactation could have baleful hereditary effects, for through the milk the nursling was still very much a part of the mother and was sensitive to any changes that might alter the quality of her milk. (Searching for an appropriate and realistic standard, Alcott suggested that the beginnings of dentition might serve as a useful point after which sexual intercourse could be resumed.) Alcott warned repeatedly that the ultimate consequences of sexual imprudence were hereditary, that the sins of one generation could manifest themselves even beyond the third and fourth generation.

In addition to Alcott's pervasive if ambiguous secularism, there is an even more mundane irony apparent in his book. Most American males simply did not order their personal lives in terms of Alcott's moral guidelines. "Young men may laugh at all this," he notes plaintively in mid-jeremiad; and indeed they may well have. Sexual behavior was still felt by many ordinary Americans to be somehow outside the control of man's conscious volition. Men still felt that the exhibition of sexual vigor was more important than chastity; many parents still laughed at masturbation in their young sons, saying—as Alcott noted in shocked tones—that it was only natural. Indeed, Alcott himself could never quite escape these traditional masculine values. Sex itself he always praised as a gift of God, a necessity for the preservation of the species; and sexual vigor he necessarily admired as a sign of health. Thus the emotional logic inherent in his plaintive intellectual distinction between sexual "power," which he could only characterize as healthy and admirable, and "excitability," which he saw as pathological, as tainted by loss of control. The historian's assumption that sexual repression and inner conflict characterized Victorian England

and America may well be based more on the defensively didactic formulations of men such as Alcott than on behavioral reality.

Charles E. Rosenberg
University of Pennsylvania
October, 1972

THE

PHYSIOLOGY OF MARRIAGE.

BY

WILLIAM A. ALCOTT, M.D.,

AUTHOR OF "THE HOUSE I LIVE IN," ETC.

Twenty-Seventh Thousand.

BOSTON:
DINSMOOR AND COMPANY.
1866.

Entered, according to Act of Congress, in the year 1866,

BY DINSMOOR & COMPANY,

In the Clerk's Office of the District Court of the District of Massachusetts.

CONTENTS.

PREFACE.................................. 5

CHAPTER I.
THE TRUE RELATION OF THE SEXES......... 7

CHAPTER II.
PREMATURE MARRIAGE, AND ITS CONSEQUENCES 20

CHAPTER III.
ERRORS OF EDUCATION..................... 32

CHAPTER IV.
ERRORS OF COURTSHIP..................... 48

CHAPTER V.
INDIVIDUAL TRANSGRESSION AND ITS PENALTIES 61

CHAPTER VI.
SOCIAL ERRORS AND THEIR PUNISHMENT..... 97

CHAPTER VII.
THE PHYSICAL LAWS OF MARRIAGE.......... 111

CHAPTER VIII.
A Fundamental Error.................. 128

CHAPTER IX.
The Laws of Pregnancy................ 143

CHAPTER X.
Crimes without a Name................ 178

CHAPTER XI.
The Laws of Lactation................ 193

CHAPTER XII.
Crimes that deserve no Name 200

CHAPTER XIII.
Directions to Parents and Guardians.... 209

CHAPTER XIV.
General Directions 246
Appendix A 256

PREFACE.

In presenting to the public a new work on an old subject, I trust I am not so self-inflated as to suppose, for one moment, that everything it contains will be regarded as original. With a few of the ideas, no doubt, some of my readers will be found already familiar. Still there are portions of the work which claim and deserve, the merit of originality.

To the publication of such a work I know of but one general objection which the wise will be likely to urge. It is that one or two of its chapters are not so well adapted to the wants of mere boys, as to those of youth and young men; while the former will be most eager to read them. The proper reply to such an objection — specious as it seems to be — is that the field is pre-occupied. If it were desirable to keep boys, for a few years, in ignorance on the subjects alluded to, it could not be done. Satan already has his emissaries abroad, in various shapes; and they are as active as if they were employed in a more worthy cause. What is left to the friends of God and humanity, as it appears to me, is to counteract his plans, by extending the domain of conscience over that part of the Divine Temple which has too often been supposed not to be under law, but to be the creature of blind instinct, in which we are only on a par with the beasts that perish.

Till within a very short time it has been my custom to exclude boys who were under fifteen years of age from my instructions on this subject. But such testimonials as the following, which is part of a letter from a worthy clergyman of New England, have led me to review my former decisions, and to change in some measure both my views and my practice.

"Go on, my dear Sir," says he, "in the good work, in which you are engaged, but do not exclude boys under fifteen years from your instructions. I am sure that at the age of ten, or at least of twelve, I could have understood and appreciated a book or a lecture on this subject."

The writer would present few claims, however, to public favor; nor would he indulge in many expectations. If he has aught of which to boast, or which should obligate the world to give heed to his words, it is his long and abundant experience among the young. He has probably attempted to guide a greater number of erring young men during the last half century than any living individual in this country. And this work to young men may be regarded as a farewell, if not as a dying legacy.

Go forth, then, little book, and fulfil thy mission. A more important post of honor, whatever some may think, could scarcely be assigned thee. May thy success be equal to the world's necessities!

THE AUTHOR.

September, 1855.

THE

PHYSIOLOGY OF MARRIAGE.

CHAPTER I.

THE TRUE RELATION OF THE SEXES.

MAN, by the Divine constitution, is a social being. It might have been ordered otherwise. Instead of being a mere individual, in a family numbering a thousand millions, he might have been made "sole monarch," of all his eye could survey. The earth we inhabit, though small among the brotherhood of worlds, bearing the Divine imprint, is yet large enough to give to each of its existing inhabitants a dividend of one hundred acres or more. How easy it would have been for Him who formed this ponderous orb of ours, to have rolled it into a thousand millions of smaller orbs! Then, after placing on each its man or woman, how easily could he have set them to revolving in infinite space, leaving the occupant of each, whether man, woman or child, to be emperor, king, president, prince, or priest of his little domain, not seventy or eighty years merely, the common age of man, but, had he willed it so, seventy or eighty million of years! And there, enthroned in all his miniature majesty, though without the pleasures that spring from an interchange of feeling resulting from the relation and feeling of husband, wife, parent, child, brother, sister, friend and neighbor, he might have enjoyed his patrimony, unenvied and unenvying. There would have been no neighbor's groves or fields or blocks of buildings contiguous to his, to excite his envy or his covetousness; nor any neighbor's children, or domestics, or domestic animals to annoy him. Nor could there have been any wars, foreign or domestic — wars of aggression or of defence — in a world occupied by only one person, and he at the same time czar, sultan, king, emperor, lord, tenant, master and subject.

Thus, I say, it might have been — such a state of things is conceivable. But God has ordered it otherwise. We are constituted essentially, one family ; with one common interest. We are so far dependent on one another, that what is for the good of an individual, on the whole, and in the end, is for the good of each and all. There are no clashing or discordant interests — there *can* be none. It is ignorance that sometimes makes us think otherwise. When I wrong my neighbor — and my fellow being, everywhere, is a neighbor, — I wrong myself. And when I do not accomplish all the good I have it in my power to accomplish for my neighbor — whether that neighbor is one mile or ten thousand miles distant — I leave, unattained, a portion of that happiness which God, in his providence, had designed for my enjoyment.

This mutual relation, and common or family interest,

will we but open our eyes, is more and more clearly perceived every day we live. The progress of the sciences — geography, history, astronomy, geology, chemistry, physiology — make it manifest. It is seen in the progress of the arts — in mechanism, railroads, steamboats and the electro-magnetic telegraph. But Revelation has always taught it. In the fullest, boldest relief, it stands, as it were, on every page of the Bible, from Genesis to Revelation. The good Samaritan was no more the brother of the wounded Jew, nor under greater obligation to love his neighbor as himself, than was Cain to love and succor and be the keeper of Abel.

But if we are to love and even to *keep* our neighbor, *in general* — if all our interests as a race, are bound up together — it is so, *in particular*. The greater *must* include the less — the collective, the individual. If, in wronging my brother — nay, if in not *keeping* him to the full extent of my power—though he be African, Indian, or Malay — I am inevitably and always blameworthy, how much greater must be the crime of not keeping, and even of not developing, in the highest possible degree, all the excellences of my nearest relatives, especially the children of my own father and mother!

By the constitution of the human family, Divine providence has laid a solid and substantial foundation or basis for the social edifice. This constitution of things, if not as old as the world, is almost so. It was one of the first decrees of the great Creator. And not until the individual and the smaller family are what they ought to be — not until of *twain* is made, as it were one flesh — is the Divine intention fulfilled or executed. Moreover, let me say, in passing, that as is the smaller family, so, in general, must be the larger one, the church; and the still larger one, the world.

In a true Christian family — arranged on the Divine plan — every one is, like Cain, constituted as a keeper of all the rest. "To thee" said Jehovah to Cain, "shall be his (Abel's) desire, and thou shalt rule over him." To him, from day to day, and perhaps from hour to hour, desires were to be made known; and by him, authority was to be exercised. More than even this is true of the divine brotherhood, that began in Cain and Abel. Each member of the family rules every other, or should do so. Especially do the elder and stronger rule the younger and weaker. This ruling, of course, is not with a rod of iron, nor even with the usual mandates of authority, but in the same spirit which Adam was required to manifest, in ruling over Eve, as well as over other and inferior beings. The language, in both instances, is exactly the same; and thus the Bible is, in this respect, as in a thousand others, its best commentator. All, whether as husband and wife, parent and child, brethren and sisters, are to do all they can for one another; and, if need be, to die for one another. They are, in all the circumstances of life, to seek each other's holiness, usefulness and happiness.

It is affecting to behold — for the scene has occasionally been witnessed — a true family; one established and conducted on the Divine basis. No one seeks his own, to the exclusion of another's good; but on the contrary, in lowliness of mind, each esteems the others better than himself. Is there a privation to be undergone? Each prefers to bear the burden, if, by so doing, the rest can be excused or exempted. Is a favor to be received of such a nature that it can be accepted or *enjoyed* by one person only? Every true brother prefers that another should receive it, rather than himself. The amount is this; they love one another, and, so far as it goes, they are based on the gospel or Christian plan. They may or may not love God, in compliance with the requirements of the *first table* of the decalogue; but they love their neighbor, according to the *second;* at least within the precincts of the family circle.

In this truly Christian state of things — where there are no Jews, Greeks, Barbarians, Scythians, bond, free, male or female — brothers and sisters, of course, exercise a very marked, and withal very peculiar influence on each other. And the influence of each on the other in the formation of character — in what might be called their education, respectively — is of unspeakable value. It is, of course, different from that of the parents, and yet, scarcely if at all less important — some, indeed, think it more so.

Boys, mere boys, and even young men, uninfluenced by the other sex, are coarse and sensual; girls, and even young women, are delicate and sensitive, but social. It is not so easy to say on which sex the influences of the other are most needed, in a case where a reciprocal influence is indispensable. The sister is hardly more necessary to the brother, than the brother to the sister.

Did these sacred, hallowed, family influences continue, the Divine plan with regard to a single generation, considered as independent of every other, might end here. The family would prepare its members for the church or the higher family; as that does for the world, present and future. "There is no school like the family school." There is no place, below the sun, which, like it, educates us — the church itself not excepted.

In the usual course of things, however, a time arrives when the education of the family almost ceases. Boys, if not girls, in their fancied wisdom and strength, grow impatient of parental restraint, and are more or less ungovernable. The passions become strong, or at least active; and so do the appetites. Just, too, at this very period — this stormy period — this Terra del Fuego of human life, the young in the usual course of things are to be scattered abroad. One goes here; another goes there. This separation of the sexes, occurring at the time when it does, what shall prevent a most inevitable and fatal shipwreck?

The ways and plans of God, most happily, are all perfect. At this critical period — though not equally so, perhaps, to both sexes — it is wisely ordered that a new passion shall spring up, unfelt or almost unfelt before. It is the love of the opposite sex. It is not exactly the love of brothers and sisters *for* brethren and sisters, though it *includes* the latter. It is much more. It is a revival or renewal of the family love, with something superadded. It is stronger than the former, and seems, in many instances, to be stronger than death itself. * Its leading design is to secure a brother or sister as a help-meet — an educator — not for a few years, merely, but for life, be that life longer or shorter; be it fifty years, a hundred years, or a thousand.

Out of this attachment, as its grand consummation, comes marriage; and hence, I again say, one of the great ends to be secured, by this most blessed institution. Or to express the idea, in as few words as possible, it is designed to complete the education of the parties — to form a brotherhood or sisterhood for life.

How wise, how benevolent the intention! If God is the author of good to the human race, in any respect — and most certainly he is so, in every particular — it is in ordaining matrimony, or a school for the final

* This statement may seem a little extravagant; but we have ample proof that it is literally and unqualifiedly true. Madame de Ossoli, in the hour of distress from shipwreck, preferred death to a separation from her husband and child; and had her choice. And I have heard many an individual express a determination — and in all sincerity too — to pursue a similar course, in similar circumstances. I do not say it is right; my object is simply to announce an important fact in the study of human character.

education, (so far, at least, as the things of this life are concerned) of the sexes.

Marriage is social and intellectual, physical and moral. Some have confounded the social with the physical — love with lust — but they are widely different. Indeed, they do not always coexist, even in our own sex; and in a normal state of things, in the *other* sex, never. Physical matrimony, sometimes prompted and frequently sustained by lust, grows out of the necessities of the case; though it seems, at first view, to be but an after thought.

It is, in this aspect of things, more particularly, that marriage becomes at once a duty and a necessity. Bad as the world now is, how much worse would it be but for matrimony? It is, so to speak of it, the golden chain that binds society together. Remove it, and you set the world ajar, if you do not drive it back to its original chaos. Remove it, and a thousand years of patient experiment would not be sufficient to find a substitute for it.*

Marriage, regarded as a duty, should be aimed at, in all our education, both of the family and elsewhere. The young, of both sexes, should be taught to look forward to it, not as a mere plaything, but as one of life's responsibilities. To marry, should be, I say, the general rule — to which, as to most general rules, there may be a few exceptions.

---

* Do not those who, in modern times would loosen the bonds of matrimony, make a most fatal mistake? It is hoped they may yet live and retrace their steps.

So indispensable has marriage been regarded by some Christian sects, as my readers well know, that it has been exalted to a religious ordinance. It is, no doubt, a religious *duty*, as much as any other; but I see no need of making it a religious *ordinance*.

It is unnecessary to stop, here, to say at what age, and under what circumstances, external and internal, this union of the sexes should be consummated. My object, in these paragraphs, is to proclaim it as a part of human duty — as a law that cannot righteously be evaded — and to show that, being regarded as a part of our duty, and as a known law, is has, attached to its violation, like other laws, its pains and penalties.

To secure almost anything valuable on earth — health, knowledge or moral excellence, — requires persevering and sometimes self-denying effort. It even requires occasionally, the overthrow of serious obstacles, or the surmounting of apparently insurmountable difficulties. It is so, with regard to matrimony; especially in an old country, and in a luxurious state of society.

Once, he who became the head of a family, secured as a general rule, a help-meet, according to the Divine intention. In the progress, not of true refinement, but of a refinement, rather, which is both unnatural and injurious, it has come to pass, as a well known fact, that in many instances he who marries and has a family, must not only subject himself to an enormous "outfit," and then be obliged to sustain himself and his children, but must maintain a delicate, feeble, or sickly wife into the bargain.

Now if all our young men had fortunes at command, this need not be set down as a serious obstacle to marriage. But to him who begins life by himself, at twenty-one, with no help but his own hands, and works for one or two dollars a day, it is a difficulty of considerable magnitude. How is it possible for a young man, in these circumstances, to marry early, and support a family, wife and all, by the mere labor of his own hands?

In saying this, I intend no reproach of female delicacy and debility; very far from it. It may possibly appear, in the progress of the following chapters, that this very delicacy and inefficiency are chargeable, in no stinted degree, on our own sex. But as to facts, I must state them just as they are.

There is also an apparent difficulty which exists even in the case of young mothers who are really healthy. Some of them are beginning to think a great deal of the proper education of their children, and a few of them actually expend so much time in this work as leaves them little opportunity or strength for anything else. In these circumstances, a young man who was not well informed, might feel, at first, as though his wife was a very unprofitable one. Indeed in measuring everything by his own standard, that standard being allowed to be perfect, would she not be so?

What, then, is to be done; and how is this difficulty to be met and overcome? I know of no other way, except by a compromise. If the cultivation of the mind and heart are deemed of greater worth than luxuries, by the wife, and if both cannot be afforded, the husband must be contented to deny himself that which is admitted to be of inferior value, for the sake of what is of greater worth. One fourth, one third, and in some instances nearly one half the expenditures of a modern family are for things which, when compared with the formation of good habits and character, in the children, by the mother, sink almost to insignificance.

But I will not, now, extend the list of difficulties. There can be very little doubt that if among the motives that impel our sex to marriage, appetite were not included, celibacy would be vastly more common than it now is. In all countries, as luxury advances, celibacy keeps pace with it. For the general truth of this statement we need not go farther than London or Paris; or even than New York.

To prevent the world therefore, — I mean of course the civilized world — from going into downright and irrecoverable celibacy, despite of known duty and final interest, that love of the female sex, to which I have referred, is sustained by a new and most imperious appetite; one which, like fire and many other potent agencies, though a good servant, often becomes a hard master.

This appetite, like the other appetites, gives us efficiency of character — impelling us forward in some direction or other — just as the heavy mall, by its physical force, impels the wedge which is before it. But the appetites are as blind as the mall itself is, and, unless properly directed by reason and conscience, as likely to go wrong as right. It is only in the brutes to whom God has denied reason and conscience and science and the light of revelation, that appetite or instinct, is a guide. And yet, the human appetites, if rightly directed, are an occasion of adding greatly to our usefulness and happiness; and, in this point of view, the stronger they are — not indeed the more excitable, but the *stronger* — the better for us and for the race to which we belong; while if not properly directed, they serve but to accelerate our destruction.

Now I have not a doubt that this appetite, in all its native strength, is absolutely needful to impel us onward in the path of duty, and to make us avoid celibacy. Nor is it possible for me to doubt that it has this general effect, the world over. It prompts to those indulgences, which, while under the control of reason and conscience not only minister to human enjoyment, but prove an occasion of perpetuating the species. This reproduction of the species is the second great design of marriage.

This third appetite, then, like the other two, is to be regarded as a *means* rather than an *end*. And yet nothing is more common than the assumption of a prerogative, and the maintenance, for it, of a post, to which it should never aspire. In too many instances, it fills the mind of the young man, to the exclusion of almost everything else. Mental, moral, and social marriage pass, with him, as of little or no account.

Progress, the great law of our nature, as intelligent beings, is nearly or wholly lost sight of.

This perversion, monstrous as it is, sometimes exists at a very early period. But its influence as a whole is always unhappy. The mind of the young should be but little occupied with it before puberty. Better, were it possible, if it could fall five or six years behind it. It is designed, by the Creator, to come into activity at about the period of bodily maturity, and to last as long as its owner. At the age of one hundred and twenty the eye of Moses is said not to have been dim, nor his natural force to have abated.

We shall see, then, in subsequent chapters, (what has been already implied), that the third, or sexual appetite, were we not sadly miseducated, would accomplish Nature's leading designs, and conduce largely, to the happiness of all concerned — the individual himself, his family and the world. Abused, as it too often is, on the other hand, it is a source of immense evil, filling society with mourning, lamentation and woe, and drowning virtue and happiness in an ocean of tears!

CHAPTER II.

PREMATURE MARRIAGE, AND ITS CONSEQUENCES.

But marriage, though a necessary agent in the formation of character, especially social and moral marriage — and hence a duty — should not be consummated too early; while love, or the attachment of the sexes, can hardly make its appearance too soon. I care not if it springs up in the very precincts of childhood, provided, always, we have wise and careful elders, and other associates, to aid us in directing it. Some of the happiest unions ever yet consummated had their origin in an acquaintance formed in the veriest youth; perhaps in the primary school-room. Indeed, in more than one instance, a happy married life has followed the playful union of the parties at six, eight or ten years of age.

Of late it has become rather fashionable to extol early marriages; and some have proceeded to an extent, in this direction, which borders on the ridiculous. Dr. Watson, of Nashville, would have this duty attended to, by the young, as soon as they feel prompted in that direction by the passions and appetites. But if it were so that marriage could be consummated at this early period, without detriment to the offspring, it could never be so well for the parents.

It is, I know, most strenuously maintained that the offspring of elderly people have a feeble organization, and are hence more liable to disease than those of the young. But this, if true, is one of the strongest arguments against early marriages, — such early marriages, I mean, as Dr. Watson recommends, — that could possibly be advanced. It is, at least, a most powerful argument against that unlawful, or at least premature, indulgence of the sexual appetite which so enfeebles a person that by the arrival of the usual, fashionable age for marriage, he is wholly unfit to marry, and is sure to propagate a feeble or sickly race.

If this early abuse of the sexual functions and organs cannot be prevented; if by the time a young man is twenty-eight or thirty, or thirty-two, his vital energies are already fast ebbing, and his natural force beginning to abate, then I grant the necessity of early marriages, in the modern sense of that phrase and term. But I cannot believe, as yet, that the world is quite incorrigible. Let us, at least, make one more attempt to enlighten and save it.

Dr. Johnson, an eminent British writer, lays it down as an undisputed point that marriage should not be consummated till we come near to maturity; at least to maturity of body. But this physical or bodily maturity does not take place, as he says, in the male, till about twenty-eight or thirty years of age; nor, in the female, till about twenty-three or four. " On the the whole," says he, " the female should be, at least, twenty-one years of age; and the male twenty-eight."

It is certainly possible that both sexes come to maturity a little sooner in the United States than in Great Britain, and other old countries; but I believe the difference, after all, to be very trifling. Physical maturity, in the United States, does not arrive, as a general rule, sooner than the twenty-fifth or twenty-sixth year, in the male, and the twenty-first or twenty-second year in the female. It requires a long time for the bony frame to become consolidated, and all its parts fully and completely ossified — as they are, or should be, in perfect physical manhood. And who, that has at all studied human nature, will believe that mental maturity is attained at a much earlier period?

Dr. Johnson proceeds to say that for every year the female marries below the full age of twenty-one, " there will be, on an average, three years of premature decay of the corporeal fabric, and a considerable abbreviation of the usual range of human existence." Thus, if she marries at eighteen, instead of twenty-one, there will be, according to this estimate, which he insists is " a fair one," nine years of premature decay; and, if she marries at sixteen, instead of twenty-one, her physical decline will be hastened no less than fifteen years!

The disagreement between Dr. Watson, before quoted, and Dr. Johnson, is glaring; like the opposite poles. Both views cannot be true. I have not a doubt that the latter is much nearer the truth than the former. Indeed, we seem, to me, to have the proof before us, every day we live, in the continual deterioration of the race.

It might be said, and with truth, that the same premature decay must be induced upon the male, in the case of early marriage, as upon the female. Should there be doubts in the minds of any, on this point, simply because Dr. Johnson has not affirmed it, let them remember that if the female fabric is prematurely impaired, at such a rapid rate, in each generation, it cannot be long before the whole race will have descended the plane, since man is, everywhere, the offspring of woman!

That the offspring of unperverted youth, of fifteen or sixteen, in the one sex, and twelve or fourteen in the other, would in itself be preferable to that of perverted manhood and womanhood, — say at thirty or thirty-five on the one hand, and twenty-five or thirty on the other, — I have not a doubt. But are we yet reduced to the necessity of a choice between these two evils?

Suppose, however, we were. Suppose marriage were consummated at sixteen and fourteen respectively. Suppose, also, some two or three healthy and vigorous children were the result. Yet, by a law of nature, — the law alluded to by Dr. Johnson, — as irrevocable as that of the Medo-Persians, there will be a degree, greater or less, of premature physical decay of the corporeal fabric, on the part of the parents, as the consequence; and the natural duration of their lives will be considerably diminished And the tendency, in this direction, during the successive generations, will be in a geometrical ratio.

But this is not all. Admit that one half the family, in such a case, — I mean, now, the first who are born, were more healthy and vigorous than the average of the race; still, is it not probable that the other half would be proportionally feeble and imbecile? Or, if the difference were not so great as to be strikingly perceptible in the first generation, would it not be in the second or third? Deterioration there would be, there must be, somewhere; it is, in the nature of things, unavoidable.

In full array against an immature propagation of the human species is the testimony of analogy. No judicious farmer is willing his domestic animals should reproduce themselves till they have reached maturity, or nearly so; nor that his fruit trees should bear too soon. The first fruits may, indeed, be equally perfect; I have even seen them preferable to those of worn-out or consumptive trees and animals. Yet, I repeat, no wise farmer would prefer them. He would prefer to wait for a little more maturity of the parent stock.

I have sometimes wondered why the advocates of early marriage, of the Dr. Watson school, can not look forward a little further than they do. Why, what can be more plain, than that a young tree or a young heifer which, instead of bearing fruit or rearing progeny as early as possible, should be restrained from bearing for one year, would be gaining physical strength and vigor, and would attain to a greater average degree of strength, in full maturity, than if it propagated itself a year earlier? The aggregate of physical vigor, in a generation of a hundred cattle, the product of parents three years of age, would be obviously much greater than that of the same number propagated from parents at two years. And let the process of propagation from ancestors of only two years, in this case, be continued for a few successive generations, and who can doubt with regard to the results? Could there be any other than a marked deterioration? And would not similar results follow in the case of premature propagation of the human species?

May we not hope, then, that the new fangled doctrine of early marriage, — the marriage of mere boys and girls, — will be abandoned? Or, more properly, may we not hope that it will not extensively prevail? May it not be reasonably expected that this important point, like all others, will be regulated by moral and physiological *law*, rather than by caprice and fancy?

I am, however, obliged to insist on having the period of intimate and special acquaintance of the sexes begin earlier than it now usually does. I know, indeed, that a few weak mothers are sufficiently anxious, already, to have their daughters go abroad, but it is not to form life-long acquaintances; it is rather to attract attention. And, even in going abroad for mere display, they usually go masked. They do not exhibit their true native character.

The special acquaintance of the sexes should begin at puberty, or even earlier. Ten years of courtship, in some instances, are not too many. Courtship forms, practically, an intermediate school for forming character, between the infantile school, or that of brother and sister on the one hand, and the school of the family on the other.

When I say that this intermediate school for the formation of character can hardly be commenced too early, I have no reference, — not the remotest, — to the customs of night visiting, and night sitting. The former of these I would, if possible, prevent; the latter, I would positively interdict. Unrestrained and undirected, such early acquaintances may wholly defeat the purposes for which they were intended; yet, with proper direction, and under proper circumstances, as I have before said, they cannot but add greatly to the sum total of human happiness.

The wise parent should encourage rather than repel these early intimacies. Some pursue an entirely contrary course. I have known many fathers, and not a few mothers, who believed it to be alike their duty and their interest to keep the young, of different families, out of each others' society as long as possible. Instead of encouraging little friendly meetings at their dwellings respectively, in the afternoon, they seemed to think it not only silly, but a great waste of time!

The results, in the latter cases, were, that these meetings of the sexes were often crowded into the evening, continued late, and badly conducted. Or, what is vastly worse, some of them were unlawfully managed. Knowing that the parents were opposed to the whole project, the young have stolen away, and joined them without permission. How truly surprising it is that parents, of good sound sense in all other matters, cannot avoid this sad mistake with regard to the young!

For, in the first place, it is quite doubtful, to say the least, whether those who grudge the day time for amusement, actually gain anything by crowding it into the night. Nature will have her rights; and what is borrowed from the late evening hours will either be repaid by late sleeping in the morning, or by unusual dulness and inefficiency during the day. Then, secondly, the tendency to clandestine excursions, and secret or illicit amours, which is sometimes thus given, is a result more to be dreaded than the former.

The truly judicious father and mother, in the recollection that they have once been young and have felt as young people now do, will by no means be backward to encourage a proper and rational acquaintance of the sexes; especially when they are pleased with the general character of the families. They will open their houses for their reception, from time to time, and even put themselves to a little inconvenience, should it be necessary to do so, in order to accomplish their object. An afternoon, now and then, when it does not stand in the way of other duties or of their studies, they will by no means consider as too great an indulgence.

At these interviews the parents themselves may, and should, be present as much as possible; not to act the spy upon the young, of course, but to add to their happiness; and, if needful, to restrain all tendencies to excess. A few parents have the tact to govern themselves in such a manner that the young will prefer to have them present; but there are many whose presence is naturally repulsive. Those parents who preserve a juvenile turn, and attain thus to a green old age, possess many advantages, and, with the young, many recommendations.

It is because the old manifest no sympathy with the young in these matters, or, perhaps, because they grudge the time, the trouble, or the expense, that so many children and young persons either neglect or refuse to make them their confidants; or, what is still worse, act openly or covertly against their wishes and preferences. And every one knows something, at least he has heard something, about the sorrows that are wrung from many a parental heart by these departures from the course which parental fondness, but not parental wisdom, had dictated.

It is not affirmed that these social gatherings of the sexes in the afternoon should, in no case, be protracted beyond sunset. In particular cases they may, no doubt, be continued from the afternoon to the evening. Not, however, in any instance, beyond the usual hour appointed for the termination of the day, with its labors, studies, and other duties; I mean that of nine or, at most, ten o'clock. And, as a general rule, I think it better that these protracted meetings of the young should terminate as early as nine o'clock.

But, whatever may be the circumstances, whoever may be present, or, whatever the influence that surounds the company or controls it, there should be no association of these visits with late hours, seclusion or darkness. All concealment or dissimulation, as well as everything low or vulgar, should be always and forever divorced from the subject of courtship and marriage.

You may be inclined to ask what possible advantages can be derived from preferences, at fifteen or eighteen years of age, which are not to be consummated, at soonest, till twenty-two or twenty-five. They are numerous; but I shall only advert to a few of them.

1. I have already called your attention to a well-established fact, that some of the happiest marriages have been the result of acquaintances early formed. It is only necessary therefore to allude, in passing, to this advantage of early association.

2. There is, necessarily, less of what I call masking, at this early age; and in these simple, friendly family meetings less than in the ordinary circumstances of later acquaintances, without the pale of the family. In truth, it is only in this way that the young, of different families, ever can come to understand fully each others' character.

3. The moral and restraining influences of these early formed preferences can never be too highly valued. A single anecdote will show my meaning; and is worth a volume of merely dry argument.

Every one has heard of John Newton. This eminent and excellent man, at a very immature age, was employed in the African slave trade. This led him into foreign ports, and, as is usual in such cases, into temptation. But an early attachment to a young lady in England preserved him, as he says, in many an instance, from falling to a depth of vicious conduct that might have rendered him irreclaimable. In the moment of peril the thought would rush into his mind, "Should I yield to the temptation, and should she know it, what would she think of me?"

I might relate many anecdotes of similar import, but this must suffice. I might also notice several objections which are made, either by the unobserving or the unreflecting, to the general doctrine I have advanced with regard to early courtship; but they seem to have little weight. Besides, I shall have occasion hereafter, more than once, to recur incidentally to this subject; and perhaps to meet some of these very objections.

The unhappy consequences of hasty, ill-assorted marriages, by persons almost wholly unacquainted with each other, are well known. It is from the observation of such premature and ill-judged unions that marriage has been so often stigmatized as a lottery. But it is not the marriage alone of those who are strangers, or almost strangers, to each other, that is to be deprecated and avoided. The sudden or hurried union of those who, though residing in the same neighborhood, have never been but partially acquainted with each other, or who while forming an acquaintance, were practically masked, — a thing which, as I before intimated, is greatly common, — is equally productive of unhappy results, and is scarcely less to be regretted.

The custom which still so extensively prevails with the young of coming together, often under cover of the night and with *masks*, that is with an artificial dress and appearance, is of little service to those who really seek to know each others' character. In the bosom of the family, where no masking is as yet known, and where, if any where on earth, we see each other as we truly are, the case is greatly altered.

Marriage, Heaven's first social institution, not to say its most precious one, when originating and slowly ripening out of these circumstances — need I repeat it? — can hardly be called a lottery. Much less does it deserve to be called a game. It is an institution every way worthy of the name, and worthy of its great and benevolent Author. It is an institution which, imperfectly conducted though it has been, has done more to keep the world together than all other influences — the church itself not excepted.

CHAPTER III.

ERRORS OF EDUCATION.

THERE are difficulties connected with the subject of matrimony to which I have, as yet, hardly adverted. Some of them have their origin in certain mistakes of early education. These educational errors present matrimony to the young under false colors; and should, if possible, be speedily and effectually removed. A part of these errors are chargeable on parents themselves, and a part on the headstrong character of the young themselves. Let me begin with the beginning.

Among the errors of parents with regard to the education of their children, few are productive of more evil consequences than the almost universal habit of making false representations to them of the origin of our species.

Before they are spoiled by miseducation, most children have some good degree of what the phrenologists call causality. They are anxious to know the whys and wherefores of many things. Some of them are, in this respect, quite philosophic. It is greatly to be regretted that this disposition in the young — this curiosity that leads them to trace out the causes of effects — should not be duly fed and nourished, rather than repressed till it becomes stinted and dwarfish; and that, too, by those who, above all other persons in the world, are most interested in their well being. Let me particularize.

A new-born infant, for example, is introduced to the bosom of a family of children; and they are taught to regard it as a brother or a sister. Its presence and society are hailed with great joy by all present; in which, of course, the children largely participate. — Amid the general joy, curiosity is ever operative. The inquiry soon comes up, whence the little stranger originated. Is the truth told, in plain and simple terms? That were productive of far less evil than equivocation or falsehood. Is the inquirer told that he cannot understand the matter, at present; but that as soon as he is old enough, he shall be fully informed? This, as it appears to me, would be not only the more safe, but the more upright and truly honorable course.

This, however, is not the course usually pursued. He is told, on the contrary, that the doctor, or Mrs. such-an-one, brought the child. Or that the father bought it of the doctor for so much money; or, perchance, of some cart-man, who came along; or, that it was dug up in a distant forest, or quagmire, or swamp, which, it is supposed, even juvenile curiosity and penetration cannot fathom; or, in other but fewer instances, he is told that God sent it.

Such replies may sometimes satisfy, for a time; but it is seldom that the matter ends here. A species of intelligence that angels might delight to convey — which angels have even, delighted to communicate —

that "a child is born," is wafted as on "the wings of the wind," to a host of playmates; who are not often slow to put their own constructions on what seems dark, or doubtful, or intricate with regard to their origin. And even if there is not found among them all an individual more advanced in the analogies of Nature than the rest, to lead the van in discovery, there are not wanting those — in great numbers, too — who are ready to laugh at the pretended revelations of the nursery, and at him who has been credulous enough, even for a single moment, to receive them.

In any event, it usually happens that, in going out from the family into the world, even if they do not search in vain for the distant forest or swamp which is possessed of such wondrous qualities, to which they have been vainly directed, the young soon learn that they have been deceived; and that, too, by those whom, till now, they had most loved, honored, and respected. And what must be the state of that child's mind and heart whose parents (one or the other of them, perhaps both) stand before him convicted of deliberate falsehood?

Our first female parent needed to commit but one offence against Jehovah, in order to stand before the world in which we live — and perhaps, too, before the whole universe — to all ages of time, and throughout all eternity, as a fallen being. So the parent who has once been detected in falsehood, or even in prevarication or dissimulation, by his own children, has fallen from their entire confidence forever. He may, indeed, become reinstated in their good graces, *in part*, but not *wholly*.

Some may regard it as a palliation of parental guilt, that the falsehood is not a deliberate, *dark-colored* falsehood; but only one of Mrs. Opie's lies of benevolence or *white* lies. But, to the young, all lies are black enough, I assure you; and no apology or palliation will make it seem to them otherwise. The parent, I repeat, stands convicted, before the tribunal of the child's mind, of falsehood; and is more or less fallen, in his estimation, forever.

And then, again, the parental attempt at concealment has awakened and increased not merely a laudable but a prurient curiosity. It is human nature to magnify, unduly, that which it is attempted to conceal from us, especially when the concealment is practised by those whom we love. And what human nature is, in the race — that is, *generally* — we may be sure is human nature in the child. Children are not those half-senseless dolts we sometimes take them to be, unless by neglect on the one hand, or brutality on the other, we have made them such. In general, they are eagle-eyed. And they not only apprehend readily, but they have thoughts and feelings.

In the case before us, they have their thoughts — and they *think* a good deal. Their curiosity is greatly heightened, and their mental apparatus quickened, in its movements, by the concealment which is practised; and their thoughts frequently turn towards the subject which we attempt to conceal or cover up. The least circumstance — the most hasty and passing allusion to it, whether in conversation, action, or books, is quite sufficient to bring back their thoughts to what otherwise might have been unnoticed or soon forgotten.

Happy the child to whom the society of his playmates, at home and at school — of his own parents and near relatives even — does not prove to be, in this respect, "a snare, and a trap, and a stumbling-block." We are, very few of us, "wise as serpents and harmless as doves." Not only do we let fall the coarse allusion, here and there; but sometimes the still coarser, not to say grossly wicked, innuendo. I have heard things said and hinted at, in the midst of professedly Christian families, that ought not to be so much as named in decent society. This vulgarity on the one hand, and that studied concealment on the other, do much towards destroying many a young person, especially of our own sex.

The school-boy watches, with eagerness, the light-falling snow, at the approach of winter; and soon forms, from the soft yielding material a ball, which he rolls, with more or less rapidity, over the thick sward. It gains, in size, at each revolution; till, ere long, it requires the combined efforts of him and his fellows to move it. So with the concealment I have mentioned. It is, again and again, revolved in the juvenile mind, till that to which it had been so prematurely and withal so unfortunately directed, swells to giant size, and occupies a space entirely disproportioned to the age or the passing necessities of the individual.*

* I shall avail myself of the opportunity which a subsequent

Is it any wonder that, in circumstances like the foregoing, the young should seek with eagerness for information with regard to the origin of life at sources which are not always the most certain and reliable? What else, in fact, could reasonably be expected? Knowledge, the curious, inquiring mind must have — from the tree in the midst of the garden, or somewhere else — and if nothing better lies in its way, and especially if, as in days of old, Satan solicits, like our mother of old it seizes and appropriates.

I have alluded to the suggestions and temptations of the devil. Now I am not a theologian, nor predisposed to meddle with theological disquisitions or terms. And yet if there be abroad evil spirits fulfilling, like the good spirits of which the poet Milton speaks, their "aery purposes," I am quite certain they will be found exerting an influence in the matter before us. If men and devils were really in league to poison the minds of the young, from the very first, I know not how or where they could hope for better success than on forestalling our efforts and filling the mind and heart

chapter will afford of saying *what should be done*, in families, by way of preventing the evils to which I have been directing attention. My object, in this place, was merely to point the young to the true source of many things from which they may have suffered, or may still be suffering; and to aid them, both in their own recovery, and in the recovery of others whom Providence may throw upon their hands for protection or salvation. It is perfectly proper that the skilful surgeon should probe, to the bottom, a severe wound or ulcer, in order that his treatment, in the case, may be such as nature demands.

with error and impurity, within the precincts of every-day life; and, as it were, under our very eyes.

Broussais, in his treatise on physiology, lays it down as a general rule — what I suppose no one will deny — that the human secretions are all susceptible of being influenced by mere thought and feeling. For example, he says, at page 215 : "every one knows with what energy ideas of love act upon the testicles." Is it then surprising that while we are rousing into unwonted activity the childish or youthful curiosity, on a subject quite in advance of its years, and turning the thoughts into a most unnatural channel, we should, at the same time, be found developing, prematurely, that appetite and those passions and feelings which belong exclusively to later years?

I have been repeatedly applied to by parents, on behalf of children of both sexes — but more frequently of our own — of only four, five, or six years of age. They were anxious to know what could be done in the way of removing a habit at which, in such young beings, one is led almost involuntarily to shudder. I have not, it is true, always found that at this early age they had *suffered* much from their wrong habits. The danger was prospective. The parents were fearfully alarmed at thought of the evils to which they supposed these unnatural manipulations might ultimately, if not inevitably lead.

And why should they not be thus alarmed? For, if other and perhaps prior errors have gone so far as already to produce a determination of the blood, in undue quantity, to the organs of generation, to an extent which leads the mind involuntarily in that direction, and results in those childish manipulations already alluded to, how much greater will be the measure of evil when injudicious parental treatment or conversation shall give a still stronger direction to the general current? Will it not be like sowing seed on a field already prepared for vice, in comparison with only casting the same kind of seed on ground both unbroken and uncultivated?

There is a counterpart to the picture, which I have faithfully presented, of the anxious parent. There are those — perhaps they do not deserve the name of parent — who not only behold the rising indications of appetites, passions, and feelings quite in advance of the child's age, with indifference, but laugh at and even apologize for them. "Why," say they, "it is only acting out nature. We do not rebuke the lambs and calves that manifest the same sort of pre-maturity: why should we rebuke our children? They will soon outgrow it." But may we not hope that parents who err thus strangely, are few and far between? As well may Satan outgrow his character, as sensual children, by being let alone merely, outgrow their sensuality.

If we make a careful examination into these abnormal cases, as medical men would call them, I fear we shall often find an error on the part of the mother or housekeeper or other near friends, which, had it not the sanction of almost universal custom, would deserve the severest reprehension. It is true there is great reason to fear that in this matter, too, there is diabolical agency. Not solely because there is abroad a saying, and has been, time immemorial: " God sends meats, but the devil sends cooks;" but because it is so plain and certain and unmistakably a source of mischief that, were not our housekeepers and those who have the care of the physical wants of the young, made at least pur-blind by some agency or another, they could not consent to it.

The evil agency here referred to, I hardly need to say, is our modern system of cookery. All our high-seasoned viands, and most of our *made* or complicated dishes are of this description. Dr. Dunglison, who is by no means to be suspected of taking sides gratuitously against indulgences, at page 283 of his work entitled " Elements of Hygiene," after making many a dolorous complaint about what he calls " the complex condition of the culinary art," and especially about the use of eggs in combination with other food, closes his criticism by saying, in the most unqualified terms, — " Hence, every preparation of eggs and every made dish, are more or less rebellious." And Mr. S. G. Goodrich, the famous Peter Parley, in his " Fireside Education," says of " pies, cakes, and sweetmeats," that " these things are universally known to be poisoning to children; and those who give them are conscious that they are purchasing the momentary smile of satisfaction at the risk of after sickness and perhaps of incurable disease."

Now although neither Dr. Dunglison, on the one

hand, as the representative of science, nor Peter Parley on the other, as representing the hosts of plain, unsophisticated common sense, has, in just so many words, affirmed that these things tend to licentiousness, yet of the fact itself there can be no possible doubt. There is abroad, everywhere, a most unreasonable prejudice against the plainest suggestions about diet and drink, when those suggestions stand opposed, in any good degree, to our natural inclinations; and it is not at all surprising that even sensible men, like those I have quoted above, should shrink from every attempt of the writer and of others to effect a change. Yet be it remembered by all whom it may concern, that just as certainly as all made dishes, from their highly concentrated and over-stimulating qualities, are "more or less rebellious," just so certainly do they prove a source of both irritation and sensuality. It is a war in which there is no discharge.

Most of our meats have a similar tendency on the young, quite independent of their stimulating character as derived from cookery. Or rather they are rendered too stimulating by our usual methods of preserving them. This objection would not lie against flesh and fish prepared for the table without having been preserved from decomposition by salt, smoke, nitre, aromatics, etc. It is the effect of preservation to which I allude. True it is that many of our meat dishes *are* made dishes; so that on more accounts than one they are objectionable, so far at least as the young are concerned.

The demoralizing tendency of confectionary has

been understood from the first; and much has been written against it. And yet parents and friends continue to permit its use in their families. Never was there so much of it consumed as at the present day, at least in our own country; and never was its use so rapidly increasing.

But it forms no part of my purpose to dwell at length on this subject, in this place; and I must leave it for your consideration. The bare statement of facts, as having an influence to miseducate each rising generation, was indispensable. The friends of the young must know, clearly and fully, what a host of dangers beset their way, and threaten and too often accomplish their destruction.

For, as if what I have hastily referred to above were not sufficient to set in operation, under the very parental roof itself, a series of fires to scathe and burn children externally and internally, as with the flames of hell itself, they become at this very juncture exposed to fires, at the kindling of others, which, joined to the former, render their destruction still more certain than before.

There are to be found, in the world we occupy, a class of human beings who will do almost anything that promises to put money into their own pockets. They will sell alcohol, tobacco, arsenic, and in short whatever they please, even though it were ever so destructive of human happiness and life. Their frequent apology is, that they only sell what they buy; o which they sometimes append the very vulgar saying "If we buy the devil, we must sell him again." Others there are, however, who make a different plea, though quite as indefensible, viz.: "If *I* do not sell it, *somebody else* will."

It must, I think, be under the shadow of an excuse not unlike these — or of one which will no better endure the test in the great day of account — that certain monsters in human shape, not only sell, in general, but particularly to the young, that which is likely, in its results, to burn up, not only the body but the soul also. They will manufacture and sell, or cause to be manufactured and sold, or, what is nearly or quite as criminal, they will connive at the manufacture and sale of, such food for the mind and heart, as often proves a means of burning up those who partake of it, in the flames of a lower, deeper hell than any which can afflict or affect the mere house in which the soul lives.

My aim here is at the manufacture and sale, all over the land (clandestinely, of course), of such books, prints, pictures, engravings, and songs, as may be found in many an obscure and filthy pen of animals, that bear the human shape, while they scarcely deserve to be regarded as belonging to the human family. In a few instances, however, I have found these obscene and wanton publications in worthier and better hands. And yet, not long; for, like corrosive agents, they eat out, as it were, the very vitals of the vessel that holds them. No one will long remain respectable under their influence.

Very few of our plain common-sense fathers and

mothers have the remotest idea how extensively circulated and read these emissaries of Satan are. Nor have our young people, in some parts of the country (I mean in some of those quiet, old-fashioned places, where the young " mind their own business "), a better idea of this mighty evil than have parents. I do not mean to say that they are wholly ignorant of such books; but only that they are not at all aware of their abundance. If they have ever been at all acquainted with them, it is only by a hasty glance. They would almost as soon be caught purloining property or slandering their nearest neighbor, as perusing such filthy publications.

The young and the old should understand this matter, just as it is, in all its enormity. They should also understand that it is owing, in no small degree, to our errors of education, especially physical education, and perhaps more than all things else to our murderous cookery, that the present state of things exists. They should know that, as matters now are, we are preparing, in the best possible way, for glad tidings to the spirits shut up in the blackness of despair, and reserved in chains to the judgment of the great day.

If these books and pictures and engravings furnished for the young reliable information on a subject in regard to which the right kind of information is most imperiously demanded, their existence and extensive circulation would not be, to the same extent, a matter of regret. But in the first place they are often quite incorrect physiologically. At least they contain, along with their truth, such a mixture of error that it requires something more than a mere schoolboy of eight, ten, twelve or fourteen years to disentangle the two, and cast away the latter.

Then, in the second place, not a few of them have a tendency to leave on the young mind very erroneous impressions with regard to woman. They assume that she is naturally sensual, like the other sex. They endeavor to make it appear that all of female reserve and modesty is either a sheer pretence or a stroke of policy. They seem to say that were it not for the well known and well established fact that " one false step forever blasts her fame," that in falling once she falls forever, while man sometimes "emerges from the ruins of his fall—" woman would be just as sensuous as her " lord ; " and some have endeavored to prove that she would be more so. This error, egregious as it is, has derived support from another class of books of much better reputation, but of no better desert, such as here and there one of the volumes of the poets and the novelists. One of these assures us, most expressly, that " every woman is, at heart, a rake."

Now it is the very young men who have become familiar with the coarser productions of the pen, pencil, and graver, so clandestinely and wickedly published and sold by thousands, who are best prepared to swallow the licentious doctrines of Byron and his clan, and to become rooted and grounded in the faith that woman, unmasked and unrestrained by conventional circumstances, is no better nor any purer than themselves.

Is it necessary for me to say that though woman is social, eminently so, no slander can be greater than the affirmation that she is constitutionally, or by natural inclination, impure? As a general rule, with fewer exceptions than to most general rules, she is as pure as the riven snow-pile of yonder eminence; at least till perverted or seduced, either by her own sex or by ours. There are monsters of both sexes; and a monstrous woman is no less a monster than a monstrous man. Indeed nothing can be more true than that " a shameless woman is the worst of men;" for a shameless woman has it in her power to do more mischief among her own sex than any other individual.

With this qualification and exception, however, woman, I say, is naturally and constitutionally pure; and young men, instead of growing up into society with exactly the contrary opinion, should be set right. They should even be made to understand that it is both their interest and their duty to keep her so. They should be taught to regard her, everywhere, as a mother or a sister, and not merely as a woman. They should regard her as a human being, as remote from a mere plaything as themselves; and, like themselves, intended to occupy a sphere but little lower than that of angelic excellences. But how different from all this is the common estimate! How much oftener is she regarded, on the one hand, as a mere plaything; and, on the other, as our lawful and proper prey!

Instead of having it for their settled purpose to sustain and increase and preserve female worth and reputation everywhere, no less than in their own family circle, how ready are the young to surmise, sneer, vilify, and asperse! Not indeed with malice aforethought, but without any thought at all. It comes of miseducation. It comes in the various ways I have mentioned in this chapter; and in many more which I have omitted to mention. It comes of the adversary of all truth and the father of lies and slanders and defamation. It comes of the lowest pit of hell; and of that part of earth which is most contiguous to it.

CHAPTER IV.

ERRORS OF COURTSHIP.

From the general forgetfulness or ignorance of our young men of this great fundamental principle of social life, that what is for the true interest of any one human being is for the interest of all, together with the prevalence of that almost universal skepticism in regard to female virtue which was noticed, to some extent, in the preceding chapter, they are often led to a course of conduct in their intercourse with young women, of which not a few are greatly ashamed when they come to themselves, in subsequent and more truly enlightened stages of their existence, and which some would give worlds, were it in their power, to be able to blot out!

No young man, of any sense or spirit, would brook, contentedly, an insult to his own sister, the daughter of his own father and mother. In some parts of the United States, were it known, by a young man, that an individual was in the habit of attempting, by words, looks, or actions, to lower the standard of modesty in a beloved sister of his, or to blunt the keen edge of her virtuous female sensibilities, he would send him a challenge. But young men, everywhere, can and do feel that they and the human brotherhood generally are insulted, even though they do not make proposals for fighting away the insult in a duel.

But why should I feel so keenly, and resent so sternly, an abuse of my own sister, while I am guilty of passing over or conniving at a similar abuse, or perhaps repeat it, in the case of an individual who happens to be the sister of somebody else? Are we not all of one family? Are we not all brothers and sisters? Whether in greater or less degree, the loss of female modesty, in every possible case, is it not a loss to the whole sex, and to the world?

There is not a day or an hour of our lives — the most insignificant of us, of either sex — when we do not share largely and liberally in those rich blessings which have their origin in the sweet influences of female delicacy, sensibility, and modesty. And when but the smallest item is subtracted from the sum total of a commodity which at the best is never too abundant in a world like this, each of us, by the operation of a law of social life which is irrevocable, must be sharers in the loss. And are we not bound, in this point of view, to be the keepers rather than the seducers or traducers of our brethren — and of our brother, so to speak, of the female sex, as well as of our own?

And yet, in spite of all these considerations, or ignorant of their weight and desert — borne away, too, by the influence of mistaken views, and perhaps of prurient and ungovernable passions and appetites — how often, during a long period of pseudo-courtship do young men make an unrelenting attack upon that citadel of female character which they should seek rather to render, not only invulnerable, but, as it were, unassailable?

They may sometimes be inclined to apologize, and to say that they intend no evil, but are only amusing themselves, or, perhaps, experimenting. But have they a right to experiment on human character in this way — especially on *female* character? Is it safe to do so? Can one go on red hot coals and not be burnt? On this point, we might learn not a little, if we would, from the experience of Solomon of old, if not from many a smaller man than Solomon, and of later date.

Those of us who are not only aware of the influence of first steps, but of the duty of acting, everywhere, the Christ-like part of being keepers of those who are younger or feebler than ourselves, will not only avoid, with the utmost solicitude, all errors and improprieties in our intercourse with the female sex, but also, as far as possible, all temptations to such improprieties and errors. We shall even discourage all approaches to forbidden ground, especially in the case of those whose character has become slightly sullied, but is not yet wholly irretrievable.

For though woman is naturally pure — as pure as I have already represented in the previous chapter — still she is easily and largely susceptible of perversion and injury both at the hands of her own sex and ours. There are, as I have already mentioned, female seducers, as well as male; only they carry on their war against humanity in a somewhat different manner; and are, numerically, "few and far between." "Well for the race, that they are so; for they scathe and scourge, wherever they are, most fearfully.*

With such creatures, in female shape, it may possibly be your unavoidable lot to come in contact; but believe me when I say it will be advisable to keep aloof from them as much as possible. Were you to think of doing them good, the hope would be almost a forlorn one. You will rarely be able to reclaim them. In my whole life I have known but one or two such reformations.

Their fall to this depth of degradation, though often sudden, is not always so. We may sometimes discover the downward tendency, in time to justify an effort to prevent any farther declension. First steps, though always exceedingly dangerous, do not always prove irretrievable. The hand and voice of friendship may, sometimes, arrest and save. And blessed is he who is awakened and moved to the duty — nay, the necessity, in self-defence — of exerting himself in this very direction.

* They fulfil their diabolical purposes, first, by teaching solitary vice; and, secondly, by suffering themselves to be employed for the purpose of leading virtuous,— perhaps, lovely — worth to dens of prostitution and infamy; and, thirdly, they give themselves up to a life of prostitution, than which nothing is more hardening to the heart.

Young men may laugh at all this. They *have* done so; they may do so again. But the time will come, — *must* come — when their feelings, in this respect, will be changed; and they will be much more inclined to weeping than laughing. There are, in this world, *some serious things and subjects;* and I am much mistaken if this is not one of them.

If we do all we can to prevent the world from deteriorating, the causes of declension will be sufficiently numerous. And let me repeat, once for all, and let it never be forgotten, that every cause of decline, even though it were but the downward departures of a single female, must inevitably and forever react, with greater or less force, on ourselves.

It has been often believed by the young, as well as by some of those to whom the term young would hardly be applicable, — and the belief has been sanctioned, if not originated by books of supposed authority — that the results of impurity to woman, physically, whether in the solitary or social forms, are not so serious, in their consequences, as to man. It has even been maintained that there was, in her case, no injury inflicted, at all.

Now, I know of no mistake in the world greater than this. Woman's finer wrought, more susceptible, organization, receives far greater injury from sexual abuse, than our own — only the punishment is inflicted in a very different manner, and, in some instances, at a remoter period. Solomon has said: " Because sentence against an evil work is not executed speedily, therefore the heart of the sons of men is fully set in them to do evil;" and one might be almost tempted to think that, in saying thus, he had the eye of his mind directed to cases like the one in question.

So remote and apparently disconnected from the crime, is the punishment, in the present instance — at least very often — that no physiologist should be surprised that the proper relation between cause and effect, has not, by the ignorant and vicious, been recognized. The only wonder is, that physiology itself should have perpetuated so glaring an error.

This error is mentioned and dwelt upon here, because it has furnished an apology to many a young man who was but half informed in the matter, and who was, in a greater degree, destitute — perhaps reckless — of moral principle. In the belief that woman was not injured, physically, by sexual indulgence, he has been inclined to give that license to his appetites and passions, which with another and an entirely different belief, might have been, at least partially, withheld. And this license, as we shall see, hereafter, has been taken, within the pale of matrimonial life, as well as without its sacred precincts.

Fornication, I do not believe to be as common now, at least in New England, as it was a hundred years ago — I mean in proportion to the number of inhabitants. Still it is quite too common. In a more dense population, the cases which occur, may seem to be more numerous in comparison of the population, than they really are. Whether, however, the substitution of solitary for social error, augurs good to mankind, on the whole, is a point to be considered in another place. It is sufficient, for the present, if I state the evil results and tendencies of the latter, and enter my protest against it.

Were it so that during a courtship protracted, as it sometimes might profitably be, to a period of five, six, eight, or ten years, the sexes were found mutually seeking, not only to become acquainted with each other, in their true character, unmasked, but to elevate and improve each other, this part of human life could hardly fail to be one of the most important, as it is now, and ever has been one of the most interesting.

And hence one reason why I have all along insisted — and must still insist — that the mutual acquaintance of the sexes should be made, very largely, by afternoon visits, under the eye — the general eye, at least, — of parents, masters, or guardians. These afternoon parties may include more or fewer families of children; yet I cannot help believing, that if we wish to accomplish the greatest amount of good which the circumstances will admit, that number should be small. And if it were restricted to four, five, or six families, I am not sure we should sustain any loss.

I acknowledge, most cheerfully, the advantages, for all purposes of mere amusement, or for improvement in science and morals, which are sometimes derived from bringing together large numbers. We are all, to a considerable extent, creatures of sympathy; and of this natural sympathy, God is the author. Nor are we permitted, for so much as one short moment, to doubt its usefulness. But those little family meetings of the young, concerning which I have said something in another chapter, are mainly for another purpose; and the less they break in upon the usual routine of the great model school — the family — the better.

On this point I greatly wish to be understood. My remarks are by no means intended to proscribe all visits *except* those simple family gatherings which I have been recommending. Far from it. With certain restrictions they may — and I suppose *must* — be tolerated, at least occasionally. They will, however, be very indifferent opportunities for studying character. This last must be learned in the family, or no where; and happy is that arrangement which—without making us members of another family, seven, fourteen, or twenty-one years, like Jacob — gives us the best possible substitute.

You see, by the tenor of these remarks, how far I am from encouraging what has sometimes been called, by way of reproach, the *convent* system. As I have already intimated, I think the family the model of all schools, and cannot help deprecating the necessity of separating the sexes from the routine of family habits anywhere. All our schools, unless it be professional ones, should include a due proportion of males and females. To this opinion in practice, I am happy to observe a very general tendency of the public mind, at least of the more intelligent part of it.

Nor would I, willingly, be misunderstood on *another*

point. My object, in bringing the young together, unmasked, is not, I again say, to encourage them to act the spy upon each other. The whole thing should be perfectly understood, both by parents and children. I do not mean to say, that parents and children, on and by these occasions, should, mutually and collectively, *intend marriage* or even courtship, especially at first. But I do mean that parents should, in this way, make known their preferences, as well as lay a suitable foundation, if possible, for the preferences of their children. If, on a fair trial, aversion rather than attachment — or even indifference — should be the result, such changes must be made as may meet the exigency.

Every one knows what a world of woe grows out of the usual custom of leaving it to the young to form their attachments at hap-hazard; and then, when they do not choose in a manner that suits us, attempting to turn the current. The changes I propose are intended to prevent any such attempts, or any supposed necessity. They include the idea of having a mutual good understanding on the subject, between parents and children, from the very first. They are designed to prevent that which having been neglected, we would, afterward, as wise parents, gladly give the whole world to undo, or eradicate.

I have alluded to the larger party or visiting circle, on rare occasions, with a degree of approbation. And yet the larger party needs to be watched with greater care than even the afternoon private circle. All fac titious things and circumstances must be removed. Conversation which is too exciting, and the presence and perusal of highly exciting books, are little less injurious than unreasonable and unnecessary heat, impure air, exciting drinks, and rich delicacies.

Any of these, however, especially the last, are made much worse, in their effects, by being taken at unseasonable hours. For, if hot tea and coffee, and high-seasoned food, and aromatics, and perfumes, and hot and impure air — with which, perhaps, music is conjoined, vocal and instrumental — are always of doubtful tendency to the cause of moral purity, how much is their danger augmented, when the party is protracted beyond the hours of nine or ten o'clock at night — perhaps to midnight, or still later? The reader will see, herein, some of the reasons why I would have no connection between courtship and marriage, and solitary or nightly visits; and, above all, night-sitting.

Yet let it never be forgotten that the society of the sexes must be cared for and properly maintained, in some shape or other, both within and without the pale of the family. The social law is God's law, from the first. "It is not good for man to be alone," is a decree that went out from Jehovah's throne, almost as soon as the human race was created; and to disregard it is to render us obnoxious to many pains and penalties. Nor has it, as a law or decree, ever yet been abrogated or repealed. And who does not know to what narrowness and selfishness celibacy tends? Who that has lived long in the world can be ignorant of the general fact that it is but a pathway to demoralization and consequent destruction?

Let all our children, then, be trained for marriage; but let it be that marriage which an inspired Apostle says is "honorable." It is not the mere union of one division or part of our complex nature — it is not physical marriage alone, nor mental marriage alone, nor even social marriage alone, important as that is. It is a union of the whole nature, in such a manner that of two we become one. As the Scriptures say, being twain we become one flesh. It is not a temporary union — a union which may be dissolved, at pleasure, by the parties; it is a union for life. It is of Divine appointment; and what God has joined together, let not man put asunder.

But by training the young for marriage, I do not mean that we should give them the kind of training they generally receive at our hands. The less of this the better. If nothing can be done with the young in relation to this subject but to excite their curiosity and pruriency, then, for anything I can at present see, the world must despair, and must ere long commence — if it has not done it already — a retrograde movement.

It is a most miserable state of things when all the teaching on marriage which the young receive, in the family, consists in reading over the hymeneal list in the newspaper, and commenting on it, and in talking over the circumstances of the latest marriages in the neighborhood. I do not say that these things should be excluded from the social circle; but only that they should not be its Alpha and Omega — its beginning and end — its all in all.

Wealth, rank, beauty, and accomplishments are not of course to be despised — they have their value. But how contemptible it is, that many, not to say most, of our best Christian families never give the young any other instruction with regard to courtship and marriage than what may be accidentally gathered from a few desultory conversations about these mere externals? What one party or the other has gained, or is likely to gain, of personal or pecuniary advantages, will be far more likely to elicit attention in almost any social circle, either within the family pale, or beyond it, than the more important inquiry whether the parties, by their union, have, either of them, increased their means of usefulness. Who does not know what is meant — and how much — by the practical and, I had almost said, only question ever asked in these cases, viz.: Has she married *well?* Are they *pleasantly situated?*

Nothing is more natural than for those parents who have just become awakened to the importance of giving needful instruction, on this great subject, to make the mistake of saying too much at once. The young do not want homilies or sermons. What they most need — what, in truth, they are hungering and thirsting and starving and dying for the want of — is just such practical every day instruction, with regard to the great end and object of married life, as they are wont to give in relation to other matters. Here they enlighten, by little and little, as the young are able to bear it; and as their minds are in an inquiring frame. Why should it not be done there, as well as here? When will the children of light become as wise, in their generation, as the children of this world?

CHAPTER V.

INDIVIDUAL TRANSGRESSION AND ITS PENALTIES.

It is a fundamental law of the great Jehovah's kingdom that as we sow, so we must reap. It is so, at least, in every instance where Jehovah has not chosen, of himself, to depart from his ordinary course of government, and make special provision to the contrary. Nor can his special dealings, of this sort, ever be calculated on. What has happened only once or twice in six thousand years, can never be properly construed into a general rule.

It is true that punishment—both for moral and physical delinquency — is sometimes very long deferred. I have seen men who worked amid the fumes of lead, who though well aware of the danger of breathing this poison, believed themselves exceptions to the general rule. They were confident that though others were apt to suffer, they should not. They had been exposed for several years, already, they said; and there were, as yet, no signs of injury. Some, however, on the other hand, confessed they were beginning to suffer slightly; but they hoped their sufferings would not be very severe; for the duty they owed to their families rendered it quite necessary that they should remain as long as possible in their employment.

I have watched the results, in both these cases. The former class, notwithstanding their supposed *imperviousness*, held out longer than the latter; but both finally disappeared. I have never yet known an individual who was able to endure the inhalation of white lead more than five or six years. All have been obliged to leave the works or die.

The overseer of the lead-works in Roxbury, near Boston, — a Mr. Prince, of "iron constitution" — thought himself full proof against the deleterious influence to which he was daily and hourly subjected. He was not obliged to be constantly in the shop, like his men; but was much of the time in the open air. However, two years did not pass, after my last conversation with him on the subject, before all that remained of him, that would have been cognizable to the senses, was covered by the clods of the valley.

A man in Litchfield county, Conn. — a Mr. Morris — who had long been exposed to the deleterious influences of lead, began at length to have fears about the safety of his employment, and retired to a small farm. Eighteen years afterward he died with every ordinary symptom of lead colic.

A Mr. Whiting of Poultney, Vermont, a man advanced in years, died some time ago, with all the symptoms of hydrophobia; although if the disease were hydrophobia at all, it must have been the effect of a bite which he received from a dog in Farmington, Conn., twenty-eight years before.

You may say that these are remarkable cases — the results of active poisons; and may perhaps be inclined to doubt whether they at all apply to the more frequent and common transgressions of every day life. But we have other cases, innumerable, which have an every day bearing. Let me mention one:—

Rev. Mr. Woodbridge, then of Hartford, Conn., and not far from seventy years of age, was beginning to be troubled with paralytic complaints, rheumatism, etc. His son, the geographer, believed his trouble arose, in part, from his very free use of coffee; but could not for some time, persuade him to abstain from it. He had used it forty years, he said, and he did not believe it had ever injured him. He at length consented to abstain from all drinks but water, and to make cold applications to his lame knee, and in a few weeks he entirely recovered. Nor did the difficulties, so far as I know, ever return.

Now it is not the fumes of lead, or the virus of the mad dog, or the narcotic effects of coffee, at which I aim, in particular, in these remarks. What I would do, is to impress upon the minds of the young, that punishment, however long deferred, must certainly come. And yet there are thousands and tens of thousands who do not practically believe it; and many more millions who never thought anything, at all, about it; although Solomon, more than three thousand years ago, seems to have understood the matter and to have uttered his notes of warning, as we have already seen.

It should, moreover, be distinctly understood that the punishment will come just as certainly when we sin in ignorance, as if we sin with our eyes open. Nor is there any atonement for physical transgression. May we not be thankful — ought we not to be — that provisions of this sort are made anywhere?

But if it were possible to escape the pains and penalties attached to other transgressions of physical law, one thing is made obvious to every day's experience and observation, viz, that we cannot escape the penalties due to transgressions of the law which concerns our appetites. Here, emphatically, the soul that sins must die. Moreover it is in relation to the laws of appetite, in particular, that the sins of parents are visited upon those who come after them.

The appetites are given us, as has repeatedly been said, for our gratification, at least in part; and when not abused they do thus minister. It is no dictate of Christianity, or sound sense, that we should set about eradicating them, as certain individuals have done, all the way, from Origen, down to the present time. Indeed we are seldom too much impelled by appetite, unless that appetite is factitious rather than normal. As I have, before, more than intimated, it seems to me that man carries weight and energy with him just in proportion to the strength of his appetites; though I admit that his energies may be directed to unworthy and ignoble as well as to glorious ends. Appetite, in short, is the fulcrum on which the lever is yet to be placed which shall raise the world. Is it not meet that the same agencies which sunk the world should be employed to lift it up again?

But although our appetites, rightly directed, could hardly, if ever, be too strong, they may become too excitable. Excitability is very far from being synonymous with strength. On the contrary it is usually the result of weakness or delicacy of constitution. When the pulse, in the adult, instead of beating sixty or seventy times a minute, rises to seventy or eighty or ninety, the excitability of the system is increased, while its actual strength is in nearly the same proportion, diminished. So, when, instead of drinking a few times in twenty-four hours, a reasonable quantity and with a good degree of thirst, we are almost constantly sipping, it does not indicate strength, but weakness, in this appetite. And so, too, of those who instead of one, two, or three meals a day, are eating as it were all day long. They give evidence of a weakened state of the appetite for food, if not even of a diseased one.

Nor do they secure the most of *animal enjoyment* who are in the habit of eating a dozen or twenty times a day, or who gratify any of the appetites too frequently. They may, indeed, think otherwise. Many thousands make this very mistake. Some of our mothers and housekeepers seem to have attained to a glimpse of truth on this subject, when occasionally we hear them tell their children and dependents that by eating their fruit, nuts, cakes, seeds, confectionery, etc., when they chance to feel an inclination, they will spoil their appetite, especially for the next meal.

Few things are more common among children and young persons — to say nothing of the habits of many who are older — than this error. In truth, so general is the custom of swallowing something of the nutritious kind, either solid or liquid, between our meals, that very few persons come to the regularly set table with the appetite wholly unimpaired. Three regular meals a day, for adults, even though they should be scanty ones, are the most which can be taken, by any healthy person, and yet preserve, at the same time, a good and healthy appetite. Indeed there is much room for suspicion that the far greater part of mankind would be far better served — and would in the same way *enjoy* more — by two.

The general principles involved in the foregoing paragraphs are applicable to the sexual appetite, with its indulgences. If we pursue the course indicated by its Divine author, it not only accomplishes its precise purposes, but ministers like the other appetites, to human enjoyment. But when we violate the laws which are connected with the indulgence of this appetite, whether in one way or another, we may and do increase its excitability, while we diminish its strength, in the same proportion. We may, indeed, in this way, increase its clamor for gratification, but we gradually extinguish our capabilities of enjoyment. But the more we yield to these clamorous demands — whether, I again say, in one form or another — the more, with absolute certainty, we increase that excitability in which they have their origin.

My remarks, unintentionally, may have left, on some reader's mind, the impression that it makes little or no difference whether the indulgence of the sexual appetite be in one form or another. But this is not exactly so. What I intended to affirm was, that the rule or principle I was endeavoring to enforce or explain, was alike *applicable* to all the various forms of indulgence, even when the degrees of excess or abuse are very nearly equal.

Solitary indulgence, so far as the individual is concerned who practises it, whether male or female, is most undoubtedly followed by greater injury, near or remote, — especially physical injury — than social; nay it is so, in its effects on posterity. And every form of indulgence, as we have already seen, and as I shall show more fully and clearly hereafter, is more injurious before, than after the period of maturity. It may not be easy to explain why it is that solitary vice is more injurious to the individual and to the race, than social. Indeed I have heard many good men object to the utterance of this same sentiment in the little book called the " Young Man's Guide." Fornication has, there, it is said, an apology. But it is not so. The writer goes as strongly against social vice, as any man; only he still insists that bad as it may be, solitary vice, or, as it is usually called, of late, masturbation, is still worse.

One prominent or rather one general reason for this

belief is found in the well known fact that solitary vice is more unnatural than social. It is a greater act of violence on life's citadel. In that form of social vice called sodomy it is indeed equally unnatural; and if possible, still more revolting. But I would fain hope, this abomination is as yet but little known, or practised in this country, beyond our dungeons and prisons.

Perhaps the most complete evidence after all, of the greater ill effects of masturbation is found in the fact that it prostrates much more, the nervous and muscular apparatus; and other things and circumstances being equal, predisposes, much more, to disease, both in the individual, and in those who come after him.

Still the young who inherit comparatively strong constitutions, sometimes go on in their solitary indulgences for a time "swimmingly," especially if there be no peculiar defect or weakness transmissible by inheritance, but lying latent, as it were, or perhaps dormant; for if there is, the abuse will be sure to aggravate or to hasten it. Yet ere they are aware — even in the case of the strongest — both their strength and their excitability begin to give way; and they pass, with great rapidity, through mania, into downright idiocy, and into partial or complete impotence.

Instead of living on to seventy, or one hundred years, in full vigor and with full strength of appetite, or like Moses, to one hundred and twenty, they often arrive at a disability of enjoyment, at least from the *third* appetite, at thirty-five or forty years, and are, at this comparatively premature period, old men — their animal juices, as it were exhausted or dried up. They have run their course, and by grasping too eagerly for enjoyment, have failed to enjoy as much, in the aggregate, as if they had made a wiser choice; and have been losers for this life and the life which is to come.

Young men of fifteen or sixteen years, on finding themselves in possession of new powers of enjoyment, easily flatter themselves that, however it may be with *others*, they are in no danger of impairing those powers. What ardently we wish, we soon believe. And what, in the ardor of youth, we honestly believe, we are eloquent to defend.

And their reasoning is specious. God has given us the appetite, say they, and the means of its gratification; but why so, if it is not to be indulged? Perhaps they have a smattering of such knowledge as some of the books and schools have been wont to teach, and have called it physiology. As the existence of the tears, saliva, pancreatic juice, etc., with the curious machinery which forms them, imply an object to be accomplished, say they, why should not the existence of a fluid in the testicles, with the accompanying machinery for its formation or secretion, imply an object, too? In other words, as the existence of the saliva, gastric juice, etc., prove that we ought to eat, why do not the existence of the genitals and their accompanying secretion prove that these organs ought to be occasionally exercised?

But there is a difference between the two. All the fluids connected with the apparatus for the digestion of our food, have for their object the well being of the individual and the continuance of his existence. The seminal fluid and its machinery on the contrary have nothing to do, directly, with sustaining the life and health of the individual. There are even not wanting in the records of men and things, facts which go far towards proving that the life and health of an individual considered without reference to his duties or relations to others, would be quite as well sustained without any indulgence of the sexual propensity, as *with* that indulgence, even though it were in the greatest moderation. It is not, indeed, certain that such a restricted indulgence as is barely necessary for the continuance of the species, does not subtract, in some degree, from the sum total of the vital forces, which God, in our constitution has meted out to us.

Much has been said, I know, to prove the healthfulness of matrimony. It must be obvious, however, that all this is merely comparative; and that the comparison is made not with a celibacy of purity in thought, word, deed, and feeling, but with one that is more or less of the opposite character. That marriage, even with all its abuses, tends, as a general rule, more to health and longevity than celibacy, with its abuses, I do not doubt in the least; and, hence, as the world now is, it must be regarded as highly desirable, were it only on the score of general health.

Were we to make the comparison, however, between

the married state as it now is, with that measure of contentment, quiet, and subordination of the passions and appetites which usually accompanies it, and a pure and virtuous celibacy accompanied by the same contentment, quiet, and self-subjection, and with the same opportunities (were this possible), for the cultivation of the intellectual, social, and moral powers, it might somewhat modify our conclusions. If Sir Isaac Newton, and Dr. Fothergill were as healthy and long-lived notwithstanding their entire freedom, during their whole existence, from every degree and form of sexual indulgence, as historians tell us they were, it does not seem very probable they were sufferers, in any considerable degree at least, mentally and physically, from their celibacy.

The reader will not, of course, understand me as reasoning against marriage, in the abstract; especially as I have already insisted on it as a primary duty. My only object is to show the fallacy of that reasoning, if it deserves the name, to which the young so often resort, which, after all, proves nothing but our aptness and facility for inventing pretexts and excuses, as Franklin would say, for whatever we have an inclination to do.

It is equally unquestionable, moreover, that God has, in the nature and constitution of things, set a limit to the indulgence of the sexual appetite somewhere short of our ability to gratify it. He has done so with the other appetites; why should he not with this? He has moreover so ordered it that, if we pass this limit, we and the whole race, so far as we are connected at all with the coming generations, are in a greater or less degree sufferers. But the usual argument of the young, which I have been combating, specious and plausible and agreeable as it may seem, takes no notice of any such limit. It goes upon the assumption that man may do what he has the capability of doing. It amounts, in short, to a kind of special pleading, and to nothing more.

The natural limit which God has assigned to the gratification of the sexual appetite must certainly be passed when that appetite is indulged in such a manner as to prevent the full development of all our powers, physical, mental, and moral; or as to cripple or embarrass them after they have been developed. It is passed, also, when we gratify them socially, at the expense of the energies of the other sex, as well as when we do so in such a way that, by the law of hereditary descent, we transmit a feebler degree of vitality, than otherwise we might, to coming generations.

Now in every instance of indulging the sexual appetite, prior to full maturity of the body, we at once retard or prevent the development of that body, and practically defraud those who are to come after us. We may, it is true, defraud ourselves and others both of the present and future generations, by wrong doing *after* maturity, but not so readily or so largely as at an earlier period.

With regard to those abuses of our systems to

which these remarks have reference, it is with premature indulgence very much as it is with premature abuses of the human system, generally. Thus, the use of tobacco, though always prejudicial to health, whatever may be the age and other circumstances of the individual, is, nevertheless, much *more* injurious, as might be seen by any careful observer, *when begun before maturity*, than when begun afterward. The downward road to vice and ill-health, at the present time, is travelled by thousands of mere boys, through the smoke of tobacco. The same remark is applicable, and with nearly the same force, to the use of alcoholic drinks, opium, coffee, and every other extra stimulating or irritating agent. More than half the miseries that flow to mankind from rum-drinking, tobacco-using, and useless drugging and dosing, would never have existence if none of these things were practised this side of the twenty-fifth year.

True it is, and I most heartily rejoice that it is so, that if none of these abuses are practised this side the age of twenty-five or thirty, they will be far less frequently indulged in, afterwards. For we are, to a very great extent, creatures of habit; and he who has travelled the right road twenty-five years is not very likely to travel another path afterwards.

In nothing, however, is the weight and importance of the general doctrine, here inculcated, so perceptible as in the matter to which this chapter is mainly directed. This is so, because the evils of sexual indulgence, whether solitary or social, are generally much greater than has usually been supposed and because, too, the tendencies to deterioration, by hereditary transmission, have seldom if ever been fully and freely pointed out. In the last mentioned particular, the public mind is, to a most lamentable extent, in nearly a profound ignorance.

Let us attempt in the first place, as briefly as the nature of the case may permit, to delineate the evils which premature indulgence inflicts upon the individual himself. These, it is admitted, have been often pointed out. Some of them have been alluded to in the "Young Man's Guide," as well as in several other works; but twenty-five additional years of experience and observation have given to the observing medical world many new facts and thoughts on the subject.

We have already seen that premature sexual indulgence hurries on, unduly, the stream of life. It is said that, when maturity arrives at twelve or fourteen instead of twenty or twenty-five years, old age comes as much earlier in proportion. Thus, in some parts of southern India, and in northern Siberia, where mothers are seen at the age of twelve years, there are not wanting old women at thirty-five. Not only the extremes of heat and cold have influence in this case, but that precocity and excitability of the appetites, which usually accompany and follow.

In truth, premature excitement, and premature indulgence, of any sort, or of either or any of the appetites, hasten on most fearfully the wheels of life. Hence their influence is so insidious, and sometimes so circuitous as hardly to be perceptible to the unpractised observer; and hence, too, many an unsuspecting young man is deceived. Possessed, by inheritance, of a pretty strong constitution, and finding his face a little more flushed, and his animal spirits a little more readily excited and raised to "flood-tide" than usual, he is naturally led to suppose that his indulgences, instead of weakening him, are actually doing him good. This consciousness, as he regards it, together with the feelings of triumph over childhood, which accompany it, and the proud assurance that he has become *a man*, impart a strength and give an impulse which, though factitious, he actually mistakes for indications of an increase of elasticity and vigor. As to living at the expense of life, he knows nothing at all about it.

Indulgence in wine, to a certain extent and for a certain time, reddens the face; and so do many other indulgences; that of sexual appetite in solitude, among the rest. It would seem that there is a strong sympathy between the genitals and the head; for when an increased amount of blood is determined to the former, as in the case either of solitary or social indulgence, there is, most evidently, a reflex action upon the brain. Nor am I sure that when we excite the brain unduly, as by hot drinks, high-seasoned food, or violent passions, or by reading, or conversing, or thinking on subjects which make their appeal chiefly to the imagination, we may not, by a reversion of the rule, excite unduly the organs of generation. In truth, there is very little reason for doubt on this subject.

Perhaps these considerations may aid us in explaining the mystery of that unexpected fall of so many literary men of high standing, as well as not a few excellent individuals of both sexes, of less elevated intellectual powers, but possessed of an ardent and lively imagination, and endued with an unusual degree of physical sensibility. But yesterday, as it were, and none too good to do them reverence; to-day, we are only able to say of them:—

"In Caprea plunged, and dived beneath the brute."

Time immemorial, there has been in vogue a saying very much like this: "Women and wine, though they smile, they make men pine." I will not attribute it to Poor Richard, nor stop to make any criticisms. The point to which I wish to direct your attention is the fact of the *association*. Women and wine certainly produce somewhat similar effects externally; but the stimulus in both cases proves, in the end, deceptive — "it bites like a serpent, and stings like an adder."

It is particularly important to young men that this error, of supposing that what flushes the face and gives such a sudden impulse to particular organs may be permanent in its effects, should be effectually removed. They call it their experience; and experience, they say practically, is the best school-master. Now, how is it possible to convince them against the current of their own wise experience?

The task is, indeed, difficult, but not hopeless. Some few there may be found who are not so thoroughly imbued with our pseudo-republicanism as to disdain all authority; they will occasionally listen; especially to those whose age and venerable appearance are such as to remove all suspicion of sinister motives.

Let it, in the first place, be deeply impressed on the mind of every young man, especially those who count themselves so very robust, and who are sure that what they call a moderate indulgence of their appetites is doing them no harm, but is even improving their condition, that they have entered upon a much frequented path. They may be led by some unforeseen accident, or by peculiar circumstances, to diverge from it, or to turn back, and thus escape the pitfalls that lie in their way, as well as the impassable gulf that yearns at the end of it. But they have no guaranty to this effect. Hundreds of our young men, who felt as strong as they possibly can, as the records of insane hospitals, and other similar receptacles, would abundantly testify, have been alienated from reason, and conscience, and God, and shipwrecked on the sands and shoals of impotence and idiocy, who, for aught which could once have been seen, set out in life with prospects as promising as themselves.

Most young men, in these days, inherit a tendency to one disease or another; consumption, gout, apoplexy, neuralgia, scrofula or rheumatism. In some, however, the tendency is very slight, and were they to pursue a proper, or duly prescribed, course, they might pass on through life in the enjoyment of tolerable health, and reach a comparatively great age. And there are a few among us, in whom the tendency to disease is so slight, or so obscure, that we do not hesitate, in common parlance, to pronounce them healthy.

These comparatively healthy individuals, while in the pathway either of solitary or social vice, seldom, at first, encounter any serious difficulties; and they can hardly be led to apprehend danger. Perhaps they escape perceptible deterioration for years. Perhaps, too, a fortunate marriage to a sensible woman, or a somewhat unfortunate one, to a miserable invalid, for a time saves them.

But perhaps, too, a fate far different awaits them. As rum-drinking has its special disease — its specific punishment — in the form of *delirium tremens;* and as every other abusive article, such as opium, tobacco, coffee, tea, etc., has its specific disease, so, also, has sexual indulgence, especially masturbation; and that disease, in terminating, is neither more nor less than a most dreadful idiocy.

It has been said, I know, that the special and more natural termination of the path of the solitary transgressor, is mania. But this is not so. Mania, in general, is only his half-way house to the chambers of death. Signs of mental aberration beginning to appear, the transgressor is, perhaps, sent to the hospital for the insane; and very properly too. If he has not gone too far, and if the source of aberration can be stopped, he may recover. A very small proportion, only, of each hundred, are thus fortunate. In general his symptoms will, at best, be only mitigated. A small number remain as they were for a time, but finally die. Those in whom the disease can neither be cured nor arrested, proceed, more or less rapidly, to the end of their career, which is drivelling idiocy of the most hopeless kind. Some of the most conscientious and promising young men of whom New England and New York could boast, and of the best family origin, have thus gone away from earth, and earthly happiness.

Should there be a tendency in the family to insanity, that is, should there be an insane inheritance, the young man at the hospital will probably linger for some time. For, in order to understand this subject properly, it needs to be observed that the tendencies to disease from whatever cause of excitement, whether from abuses of appetite or anything else, are apt to be in the direction of previous constitutional or acquired weaknesses. Thus, if a person has a tendency, whether acquired or inherited to pulmonary consumption, masturbation, instead of bearing him down to the regions of mania and thence onward to the more doubtful and darksome world of idiocy, will hasten on the consumptive disease. So if the tendency be to the liver or any other organ, the voluntary abuses of the individual will hasten on to its final termination, or greatest height, that disease to which, previously, he was inclined.

It is, in general, only when there is no **marked**

tendency to any other disease that sexual abuses run the transgressor so readily into hopeless idiocy. If there is a tendency in the family, or in his own constitution as I said before, to insanity, the diseased tendencies may linger there a long time — perhaps till he perishes. But if the tendency is to consumption or some other disease, and especially if the tendency that way is strong, it will save him from mania and idiocy, to kill him of consumption.

It is, however, rather common for those, who, being inclined to consumption, fall early into sexual indulgences, especially solitary indulgence, to become affected with what is called, in books, *tabes dorsalis*, but which might just as well be called consumption of the back. It is a very frequent disease, of late years; and is, I think, in the increase.

On this subject — the tendency of sexual abuse to consumption — much might be said. The chapter on the law of marriage will reveal other facts of importance; and so will the chapter which furnishes counsels and directions to parents, masters and guardians. I have no more room for it, in this place.

An individual may tend, by inheritance or otherwise, to epilepsy; or, as it is vulgarly called, falling sickness. In that case, instead of becoming a victim to idiocy or mania, or consumption, his course will be to epilepsy — often of the most incurable kind. — It is worthy of remark, moreover. that a disease of any kind, whether mania, consumption or epilepsy, that might otherwise have been mild, or at least not speedily fatal, will be rendered more severe or more dangerous or both, by additional tendencies induced by sexual abuse. Particularly is this true, in the case of epilepsy. Many a young man might get along very well with his epilepsy, if he would govern his appetites, especially the *third*.

I knew one case of epilepsy quite in point, and striking. It had its origin, apparently, in blows on the head at about the age of twelve years. Masturbation, into which the young man fell three or four years afterward, greatly increased its severity. Excessive abuse of his stomach added still more to the difficulty and danger. He was cured at seventeen or eighteen years of age by entirely subduing his appetites; but he relapsed into stomach indulgences, and perished soon after of consumption.

St. Vitus's dance, or, as the books call it, chorea, is another disease which is often brought on some of our most promising young men, as the consequence of masturbation; — and a most troublesome disease it sometimes proves. It is not by any means pleasant to the sufferer himself to find his arms or legs twitching about, when he would gladly control them; and it is sometimes still more unpleasant and painful to his friends. It is, moreover, a disease which is not easily cured.

Should there be a tendency in the system to any other disease, such as palsy, apoplexy, hypochondria or hysteria, the result of sexual abuse of every kind, would be to aggravate that tendency; or if they had hitherto remained latent, in the system, to rouse them into activity.

One of the diseases last named, viz., hypochondria, is usually thought of as purely imaginary. Now though the imagination is both excited unduly, and disordered, withal, as well as excited, it is doubtless founded on diseased internal organs; especially some of those which are connected, more or less, with the function of digestion.

In this dreadful disease — more dreadful to my own mind than the small pox or the cholera — the sufferer sometimes imagines his legs to be made of glass, and supposes he cannot move an inch without breaking them. In other instances, he supposes there are animals of various kinds preying upon his very vitals. In others, still, he fancies he has enemies, secret or open, plotting his destruction, — perhaps even among his best friends.

The most dismal forebodings occasionally make a part of this strange disease; and not a few have actually committed suicide to rid themselves of an anguish which they deemed unsupportable. They are always, in appearance, downcast or shamefaced, as if they thought not only their limbs but their bodies also were transparent, and that everybody was looking through them.

And yet these patients are scarcely more hopeless of recovery than those who tend to paralysis. Neither is liable to die suddenly; but it is also true that neither is very likely to get well. The fate of the consumptive and the idiot is well known and settled; but the condition of those that are doomed to die a living death is little more enviable.

Gutta serena, sometimes called amaurosis, or a species of blindness, is by no means an unusual effect of the form of vice to which I am directing the reader's attention. Indeed all forms and degrees of sexual abuse seem to me to injure, more or less, the organ of vision.

But I repeat that any disease, whatever, to which the system is predisposed, whether induced by inheritance, or by causes applied to the individual himself, may be roused to activity or aggravated by sexual abuses in every form and degree. The most common disease — a cold or a fever — falling upon a person who, by these abuses, had irritated and agitated his nervous system (an effect which is, in these cases, always produced) is thereby rendered more troublesome, if not more fatal.

But I find I am likely to be less intelligible, in my remarks, than if I had explained, more fully and particularly, the difference between the predisposing and exciting causes of disease. Let me do so, by a very humble comparison.

Suppose a musket or a piece of artillery were to be discharged for some purpose, as at an enemy. It must first be loaded with powder and ball. But will it go off — explode — without anything else being done? Not in a thousand years. It is only *predisposed*, so to say, to go off. Before it can go off, it must be ignited, or *excited*. The powder at the bottom, must be set on fire.

But unless the powder is ignited, I say again, it would never go off. It would be merely *predisposed* to go off. Just so with regard to many of the diseases, to which, in this world, we are predisposed. The predisposition would not kill us. I had almost said it would not hurt us. Could we be so fortunate as to avoid the igniting spark — the *exciting* cause — I see no good reason why we might not pass through life predisposed to gout, mania, rheumatism, and even consumption, and yet die of old age.

Now young men should know that by their various personal transgressions of physical law — aye, and of moral law, too — at every age, saying nothing, now, about inheritance, they are *predisposing* themselves to disease of some sort. Half the world die of fevers. But there may be, and must be, a thousand predispositions, greater or smaller, to these fevers; and yet no human being could ever die, merely of these predispositions. There must be first, an *igniting spark*.

But every abuse of an appetite, where these predispositions exist, is or may be an igniting spark. In any and every event, it is an injury. If it do not ignite the pile of combustible matter, it adds to the predisposition, or loads the piece more and more, till at length whenever a more intense excitement is applied, the explosion takes place, and may be terrible. As a general rule, every abuse of the human system adds to the severity of its subsequent diseases. Of this, however, I may say more hereafter.

There is an evil connected with masturbation, on which its unhappy victims are accustomed to dwell, with peculiar emphasis. I allude to the involuntary — and chiefly nocturnal — emission of a fluid whose emissions at first, only take place in connection with voluntary effort. Few things give to this class of patients more anxiety and trouble.

Now it is the weakness and depression which immediately follow these nightly emissions which lead young men to think so much of their evil tendency. They forget — rather, they never knew — that what they call a disease, is only a symptom; an effect, but not a cause. Perhaps they are misled by the books of which I have already spoken with so much disparagement; and which contain, along with some truth, not a little error.

Tissot, for example, together with other German and French writers, has much to say of the muscular and nervous debility which results from these involuntary discharges of semen. The loss of one ounce of this fluid, so we are told, is equal to the loss of forty ounces of blood. They thus turn the mind of the criminal to the effect, rather than the cause of disease. And this opens the door, as it were, to a world of quacks, and brings, at once, upon us, a deluge of quackery.

It ought to be known, to all young men, that the loss of semen, in itself considered, is of little comparative importance. This fluid was not made, it is true, to be thrown off from the living system recklessly, any more than the saliva. Yet after all, it is the great agitation of the nervous system — it is the *wear* and *tear* of the vital powers, and the waste of the vital energies, which accompany or rather precede the discharge, and not the mere discharge of the fluid itself — which do the mischief. The weakness and depression are an effect, too, and not a cause.

Whenever young men can be properly informed on this point, they will be far less liable than they now are to fall into that unhappy state of the mind and heart, which is sometimes witnessed by the physician and friends, but which is concealed from the eye of others — a state bordering closely upon despair, and sometimes leading to it.

Even if the emissions become very frequent, there *is* nothing to be gained by mourning over them, or even by dwelling on them, in our thoughts. Dr. Rush used to assure his patients that if the emissions did not happen more than twice a week, they would not hurt them. But I do not think we are authorized to say quite as much as this. Twice a week indicates at least a bad condition of the general system — one which would justify, if it did not even require, a little anxiety.

I must not stop, in this place, to point out the proper course to be pursued by those who are already beginning to pay the fearful penalty of their physical transgressions. This, and the manifold dangers from quacks and quackery, to which the young are liable, will be more fully unfolded and more amply discussed in another chapter.

It is sufficient, for the present, if I succeed in impressing upon the youthful mind this leading idea that the danger to which, as a transgressor, he is exposed, lies chiefly in the *causes* which pave the way to nocturnal and other seminal emissions, and not in the emissions themselves; and that it is to the removal or prevention of these causes that our attention should be chiefly directed. Those effects which so fearfully agitate their minds *should* indeed so far agitate and affect them as to make them give heed to a warning so terrible. It is not nature in sackcloth and ashes, merely, it is nature giving vent to her agony in other and more unmistakable signs. The sorrows which most threaten the security of life's deep foundations, are not those which manifest themselves by a shower of tears. In the deepest earthly grief which is known, there is no weeping.

When a young man who is conscious he is pursuing a wrong path, begins to perceive his appetite to be affected, and especially to be irregular; when the work of digestion, and perhaps the performance of other functions, is accompanied by darting pains, in different parts of the body; when to these are added a dark semi-circle below the eye, a tumid upper eyelid, weak eyes and flushings of the face, with nightly emissions, let him beware of danger. If, however, to all these is added an unusual and unaccountable weakness of the back, lungs, and nervous system, accompanied by a dry cough and hurried breathing, a weak voice and great tremulousness, let him know that without reformation, speedy and effectual, a most fearful retribution cannot be far off.

I have dwelt, thus far, for the most part, on those evils which fall upon the criminal himself; and have said little of the results to those who are to come after him. Even, in the "Young Man's Guide," the first work in the United States which attempted to make the subject popular, almost as little was said. Other writers have pursued nearly the same course. Perhaps, like myself in former years, they supposed it to be a topic which would fail to excite their interest.

But my views are somewhat changed. Young men do not seem to me so reckless as older persons are apt to imagine. They are indeed thoughtless. They are, however, as ignorant as they are thoughtless; and perhaps their very thoughtlessness is the result of their ignorance, at least in not a few cases. In the matter before us, it most certainly is so.

Is it strange that our young men and young women should be ignorant of the laws of hereditary descent? Why, they are not made known, in any considerable degree, to one in ten of those who are older, and how, then, can the young, as a general rule, be expected to understand them? Such an expectation would be in the face of all experience and all observation, as well as absolutely and strangely unreasonable.

If a young man knew that by yielding to temptation and seizing what are known to be the unlawful gratifications of the present moment, he was preparing himself to become the father of a sickly family of children, would it have no influence with him? I do not ask whether it would *always* preserve him from self-immolation; but would it *never* save him? Or if it should not wholly preserve him, might it not partially? It is certainly worth the trial.

Let me say then, most distinctly, to every young man, that as surely as he shall ever become the father of a child which shall be formed in his own likeness, — that is, shall be like him in physical constitution — that child must suffer, more or less, from every abuse of his (the father's) constitution, prior to the period of his birth, but particularly during the first twenty-five years of his life.

Does any such young man wish to be roused at midnight or two o'clock to go in pursuit of a physician for his sick child? Perhaps he has been at hard work, all the preceding day, and greatly needs rest. Perhaps he is, himself, unwell, and needs the aid of "tired Nature's sweet restorer, balmy sleep." Perhaps it is exceedingly cold or stormy without, and he dreads the peltings of the snow or rain. Perhaps the distance to a physician's office is considerable. Perhaps, finally, the child is attacked with croup or cholera or convulsions, and the danger is imminent, so that he is almost unwilling to leave him.

There are a thousand other smaller difficulties, which in the aggregate amount to something, and require not a litle energy and effort. He is a young man, and keeps no horse. The case seems an urgent one; shall he delay long enough to go and procure a horse, — with a degree of uncertainty how long a time it will take to get started on his journey, — or shall he set out on foot? Shall he go for the nearer physician, whom he dislikes; or for the more remote one, whom he prefers? Shall he rouse some near neighbor from his slumbers to remain with his half-distracted companion while he is gone; or shall it be his first object to procure a physician, regardless of every thing else?

These are only indications, mere hints, painful as they may be, of what a young man is sometimes called to experience while at the head of a family. And scenes like this may have to be acted over, again and again, during many long years.

Another consideration is of too much importance to be excluded from the account. A young man who is just setting up in life, and even one who is a considerable way advanced in it, values his time highly, as well as his money. He does not like to spend his days and nights, perhaps in harvest time, with his sick children; nor to pay away the earnings of other times for attendants, medicine, and physicians; perchance, too, for grave habiliments, and coffins, and grave-diggers.

Besides, a child is practically an investment of property, to the full extent of what it costs us to raise him to a given age; and this is an item of loss which, when a child dies, — though many parents may shrink from it, — must certainly come into the general reckoning. Colored children are oftentimes valued at so many dollars and cents per head; are white children worth less than black ones? And then, finally and worst of all, and most to be dreaded, — should a child die, in the case just supposed, there is the painful, unspeakably painful task of following him to a premature grave.

Now then, I say, is a young man, for the sake of a little premature gratification, prepared to encounter all these, and many more kindred trials? Is he willing to sacrifice the future to the present? Is he willing in fewer words and better English, to gratify himself *now*, that he may slay his child and torture his own soul *in time to come?*

But I know the heartfelt response of every young man to these inquiries. Taking him as merely a selfish and instinctive being, without a particle of the love of God or his fellow man in his soul, he yet shrinks from the bare thought of pursuing a course which shall involve such results, even for a moment. Convince him that he is doing so, and would the conviction fail to have influence?

And yet is he not, in many instances, doing all this? Every indulgence, as I have before said, which is a violation of nature's laws, and especially every such indulgence before marriage, is doing this. I care not so much if it is the mere indulgence of the appetites for food and drink; still, the tendencies of our various violations of the third appetite are rather the worst.

Do not misunderstand me. I do not mean to say

that children would never have croup, or any other disease, without parental transgression. There are few diseases that owe their existence to any one cause to the entire exclusion of all others. A dozen causes, possibly a hundred, predisposing and exciting, may have their weight of influence. But I do and must insist, that no form of licentiousness is without its influence. Such a result were as impossible as for water to change its course, and run up hill.

No child, born of erring parents, and taking the peculiarities of constitution of those parents, is, in this respect wholly unaffected. Even when, for the most part, he follows in physical constitution his grandparents or even his remoter relations, he usually takes a tinge, so to call it, from his father or mother, or both.

Let me also say, still farther, that every disease which befalls a child, at any age — from a cold to the cholera — is the more severe and the less manageable, and even more likely to prove fatal, in consequence of every form and degree of parental transgression. I have even known the effects of drunkenness and licentiousness to be visited upon the third and fourth generation. The following is a case in point: —

A fine young man of New England, with a rising family, entered the army of the revolution, and after a few years became a somewhat distinguished officer. But his associates, as an officer, at length ruined him; they led him into habits of intemperance and licentiousness, in which habits he at length ended his days.

Now half his children, — for he had a considerable family, — were born before the war, and half afterward; and the difference between the posterity of the first, in their various generations, down to the fourth and fifth, and that of the second, is as marked as if they belonged to entirely different families. While most of the individuals descended from the temperate man before the war, are strong and healthy, the greater part of the other sort have for their portion, by inheritance, more or less of scrofula, consumption, rheumatism, cutaneous disease, premature decay of the teeth, etc.; and quite a number of them have not apparently lived out half the days which God and nature assigned them.

Indeed, it sometimes happens that when the causes of disease in a child fall short of producing their wonted effect, the inherited tendency, like a weight thrown into scales nearly balanced, decides the case in the diseased direction.

More than even this is true. Not only does every parental error tend to aggravate, if not to induce, disease, but it has also the effect to transmit general delicacy, if not actual debility. How many there are who drag through life, merely existing, as it were, when they might have been so many robust and healthy men and women but for this cause, namely, ancestral transgression?

Then, again, parental transgression has its effect on the mental strength and activity no less than on bodily health and vigor. We know not, and never can know till the GREAT DAY shall reveal it, how many mental, no less than bodily, weaknesses are the result of sexual abuse; saying nothing of innumerable other errors.

Indeed, I have not a doubt that, by the law of hereditary descent, many a licentious indulgence, especially before the age of twenty-five, has resulted in a greater or smaller degree of mental inactivity and imbecility; as well as in various erratic affections. We love what we ought to hate, and hate what we ought to love, as the result of heart-feebleness, so to call it; and this heart-feebleness is often chargeable on the forms of parental error, to which I have in this chapter been directing attention.

In the preceding paragraphs I have appealed solely to the young man's selfishness. I might, it is true, have appealed to a higher and nobler principle. For, if a few young men among us are to be supposed wholly selfish, it is not generally so. There is a mixture of benevolence, or, at least, of sympathy, greater or less, in almost every human being, however fallen and degraded. Mankind are not, to use a legal phrase, "all and singular, devil." I do not say that the majority of them, or indeed any considerable minority, possess the benevolence of the Gospel; but there is, in their hearts and souls, a fellow-feeling.

This feeling is so strong that it would make most of us shrink from the idea of inflicting positive wrong on any human being. I speak still of tne majority, and not of all. Not one in ten of our young men, as they come up in life, uninfluenced by out of doors depravity, would murder, rob, or openly defraud an African, an Indian, or a Malay. They would not rob him of his money. Much less would they be inclined to rob him of his reputation, health, and life.

But if they would not, in any of these various ways, injure those who are so remote from them, how much less readily would they injure those who are near and dear to them — who are, as it were, bone of their bone and flesh of their flesh?

Not a few of our young men who are at the head of their respective families, truly love their children as they love themselves. They would as soon — perhaps even sooner — inflict an injury of any sort, on themselves, as on their children and family. They suffer to their very extremities when their little ones suffer.

And yet, following out the train of reasoning above, is it not true that every young person who abuses his own system, before and during the time of his being a parent, robs his child of a measure of that vitality which God, in his wise Providence, designed for him? Fortunate, indeed, is he, if his transgressions do not prove the means of the absolute destruction of his child! Fortunate — should I not say thrice fortunate? — if he is not guilty of the still higher crime of manslaughter. Observe, however, I do not say murder, in such a case; but, simply and briefly, manslaughter.

Those young men are rarely found — whatever may be thought — who can resist the spirit of appeals like these. I repeat — young men have not been, in this particular, duly informed. Where the blame should rest — in the eye and mind of God *does* rest — it may not be easy to say; but there is error, somewhere. Perhaps it is justly chargeable on society as a whole, rather than on any particular class. If so, let it there rest.

And yet not necessarily. Society is made up of individuals — *begins* with individuals. The work of declension or deterioration must have begun with individuals; why shall not a work of reform begin there, too? Let *not* the matter rest, then. Let every young man who reads these pages, resolve, in his own mind and heart, to do all in his power to effect on society, a most important and most thorough work of reform. Shall he not, at least, take the first step — that which must, forever, be the first step — shall he not reform *himself*?

We think, sometimes, and speak of Eve — and her mighty work of declension. We speak of her fallen posterity — at the present time almost a thousand millions; saying nothing about the many thousand millions of the sleeping dead. Now, every young head of a family, for whom I write, may one day have been the progenitor of more millions than Eve yet has. And is not this a solemn thought? Is it not a thought of great and absorbing interest? Whose heart does not beat high at the bare possibility of becoming the progenitor of a world, as it were, of pure, holy, healthy, and greatly elevated beings — a race worthy of emerging from the fall — and of enstamping on it a species of immortality?

CHAPTER VI.

SOCIAL ERRORS, AND THEIR PUNISHMENT.

I HAVE already ventured the opinion that fornication is somewhat less frequent among us than it was a hundred years ago. It is an opinion to which I still adhere. Or, if the crime is as common now as it was then, I doubt whether it is quite as unblushing. — And is there not something gained to the cause of truth and righteousness when vice, instead of holding high its unblushing or impudent head, seeks retirement and concealment?

One can almost remember — one, I mean, who is at all advanced in life — the time when not only night parties, and concerts, and balls, and individual night visits, were frequent among the great mass of our people, but even night-sitting. I can certainly remember such a time. A young person was not thought to act well his part who did not participate at all, in these follies.

Bundling, as it was called, I do not remember. To those who know the human heart and the strength of temptation, it seems strange that it should ever, for one moment, have been tolerated. And yet there are remote parts of our country — especially of our eastern States — in which it but recently prevailed, at least in some degree.

But all the follies I have, thus far, in this chapter, referred to, except perhaps concerts and balls, seem to be on the wane; for which we owe much to God and an enlightened public sentiment. Night-sitting, in most places, is nearly unknown. Still there is quite enough of it; and quite too much of fornication, at least in some particular parts of our country.

I have already expressed a doubt whether masturbation, as a substitute for fornication, is a public gain. I might have said more, viz., that so far as it has beeen introduced *as* a substitute, we are losers by it. I do not think it any better than fornication, even for females themselves. I do not believe it to be half as injurious to a female, physically considered, to bear and nurse a child, every two years, as it is to practise solitary vice, during the same period of time. If matrimonial life, and the bearing and rearing of children, by being begun at the early age of sixteen, cuts off several years of valuable female life, masturbation cuts off a still greater number. And the delicacy and disease it inflicts on themselves and the next generation are to be, at the least, equally dreaded. Its effects on our own sex, that is, comparatively, I have already mentioned.

But though solitary indulgence is so bad, in its effects — one of the very worst scourges ever inflicted on the civilized world — it does not thence follow that fornication is not a great evil. As masturbation has its specific and awful penalty — a most drivelling and hopeless idiocy — so fornication has, too, its penalty, only in another form. The syphilis, or venereal disease, in its various shapes, appears to be by the appointment of Heaven, one of the safeguards of the virtue of the species; and woe to the individual who disregards it!

It is less easy to trace the disease to those parts of the world where it first made its appearance, than to ascertain how it now originates. But, however, this or any other circumstance may be connected with the disease, of one thing we may be sure, viz., that it is an infliction of high heaven — an almost direct punishment of crime.

Perhaps this foul disease is as old as the world in which we live; at least as old as the world that was drowned. In portions of the world after the flood — most certainly in the cities of the plain — social abuse, at least of the kind most revolting and abominable, was well-known. But of this I have spoken before.

Whether fornication, as well as sodomy, was common in the old world, we are, of course, ignorant. That in the days of Noah, and at the approach of the flood, "they were eating and drinking, marrying and giving in marriage" — giving themselves up as slaves to their appetites and lusts — certainly looks suspicious. Yet whether the modern penalty of social vice, among the sexes, was then inflicted, we have no means of ascertaining.

It is thought by some, that this foul disease may be

generated by social indulgence, at least in certain circumstances, without the existence of contagion or infection, or any peculiar predisposition. It certainly must begin somewhere; for it is more or less severe, everywhere, in proportion to the extent to which the abuses of the sexual system have been carried. The deeper and more loathsome the prostitution is, as in some of our most densely populated cities, the more dreadfully loathsome is this disease; but if it can be aggravated, made many fold worse by indulgence and abuse, in almost every degree, why should not the larger and more excessive degrees of indulgence actually originate it, especially when cleanliness and purity, and all the other laws of health are grossly neglected?

Of course, social indulgence weakens both parties in body and mind, and tends to bring on them and their posterity a thousand ills; such as I have mentioned in the preceding chapter as being connected with solitary vice. I need not repeat in this place what the reader can so easily turn to, and examine and reflect on for himself.

I greatly desire to present to the young, especially to young men, for whom mainly I write, a few of the horrors of venereal disease. And yet the thing is hardly possible. To do so would require that we should visit, together, some of the dens of prostitution and infamy with which portions of our highly favored, but greatly diseased, society abounds.

It would be necessary, in order to a correct knowledge on this point, to conduct a young man to the places which the inmates of our houses of ill-fame occupy by day, and let him see, in all or nearly all of its native deformity, the half putrid and highly offensive carcass that, at other times, is partly concealed by costly habiliments, forced smiles, paint, and darkness. Here would be a revelation, — to many a young man, — of what, in his ignorance of himself and human nature, he could before have hardly expected. He should also witness the temper with which the internal agonies of a being whose very bones are, as it were, consumed, are sustained.

If there is a living hell any where above the earth's surface, it is a boarding-house for prostitutes. If there are infernals not yet quite shut up to the blackness of despair forever, it is the inmates of such a house. If there is spiritual misery, without a parallel, anywhere, it is here.

To form anything approximating to a correct idea of the misery to which I allude we must take, in imagination, one journey more. We must visit together some of our medical museums. Here are specimens, in great numbers, of diseased formations in the human body, not a few of which are the result of venereal disease. Bony, as well as fleshy parts, are changed, and enlarged, and distorted to an extent of which, before, you could have had no conception.

The dreadful disease of which I am speaking is, as you already know, communicable; and, though it may sometimes be originated, it is usually acquired by contact. In some of its forms, however, it is so mild as not to be suspected from any external appearances, even the face. And yet in some of the severer cases I have met with the most dreadful inroads are made upon the throat, mouth, and nose. I have met with individuals whose noses had been literally eaten off, so as to present little if any prominence beyond the general level of the features.

The best troops, in making an attack in time of war, are usually placed in front of the army, and this for various reasons. One, is to cover up or conceal a body of men comparatively inferior, or perhaps greatly enfeebled or crippled. In a similar way, and by a similar manœuvre, many a young man has been deceived with regard to the hosts of the houses of death. The troops which form the vanguard of this numerous army are, usually, such as are comparatively healthy; or, at least, such as with the aid of rouge and dress can be made to appear so. Hence he is often deceived and lulled to security till a dart, as Solomon says, strikes through his liver, and he is reckoned among the strong men cast down, or the slain.

But there is another thing that lulls to security, in these cases, and thus facilitates the downward progress of many a young man, namely, the ease with which he supposes he can be cured of this disease, should he happen to contract it. He is told, perhaps in books of various kinds, — some of them purporting to be the productions of wise and learned professors, — that almost all our young men, sooner or later, have this disease, at least in some of its milder forms; and he is easily led to believe that, after all, it is a very trifling concern, at least if it can be kept in concealment.

Our newspapers, moreover, especially our dailies, teem with the advertisements of those who call themselves physicians, stating in the strongest terms that, for a smaller or larger sum, they can and will cure all, or nearly all, the secret ills that flesh is heir to; and, perhaps, in the short space of three days. There are papers that secure to their owners a good living by inserting such pompous and wicked assurances.

Now, I do not presume to say, that none of those who advertise in this way are, or ever were, regular physicians; but I must say to the young, — for duty compels me, — that they are wholly unworthy of the name; for, if they ever were physicians of respectability, they are now fallen ones. Satan, the prince of darkness, was once, so we are told, an angel of light.

These men know, and the public ought to know it, that if the terms, quackery and humbuggery are ever applicable, it is here. No matter, however, perhaps they think, as long as they live well on their humbuggery!

Another term, however, would be little less applicable. They have been called bloodsuckers; but this is too mild. Sharks — land-sharks, if you please, would be preferable. For if they do not quite swallow those of the young who throw themselves into their jaws, they at least swallow a large sum of their money.

I do not say that they never effect anything resembling a cure; for they certainly sometimes do. In other cases, however, and those probably the majority, they are of no manner of service. They get their fees, or at least one half, and this is usually no mean sum; and the patient is left, for the most part, nearly as he was at the beginning. Nature, however, even if the medicine is comparatively inert, will, in the meantime, often rally a little; and there will, at least to the unpractised eye, appear to be a degree of improvement. Yet as to a perfect cure, — as to effecting much more than nature, unaided, would have effected, in the same time, — I have many doubts.

In short, when once the solids and fluids of the human system have been thorougly affected by the poison of this foul disease, I do not believe they are ever again perfectly restored to their purity. Nature may, indeed, in process of time, wear it out in part, but I think not wholly. Trust her, however, and not quackery. Obey her laws, and in due time the terrible virus will work its way out of the blood, at least partially. Or if you consult medical skill at all, call in your family physician. Do not put your very life and health into the hands of a man with whom you would not trust a dollar of your money.

The young man who really desires to avoid every form of this terrible disease, and who believes tha prevention is better than cure, has before him a plain path. He has but to take heed to the old adage: "Every one should mind his own business;" and he is safe. If he avoids the first steps in this downward road, he will avoid all the subsequent ones.

Once more I entreat every young man to leave off putting trust in the skill of these boasted half conjurors. They promise more than they can do. They seldom or never, so far as I have been able to ascertain, effect a permanent cure. In nine cases of ten they do no good at all. Believe not even Professor Miraculous, of Wonderful College. His new book, though it should sell by ten thousands, will prove a broken reed, which shall pierce him that leans upon it.

A highly intelligent young man of Massachusetts told me, not long since, with great assurance, of a new book, such as is hinted at in the last paragraph; and asked me what I thought of the author's theory. He said he appeared to be a very learned man; and mentioned, in proof, his connection with a certain college. I told him I doubted, seriously, whether a gentleman of that name had ever been connected with the said college, as one of its professors; for I had known something of the college for many years, particularly the last year.

The public cannot be too much on their guard against impostors of this description. It is not long since a young man calling himself Professor C., of Andover, Massachusetts, travelled in northern Ohio, giving lectures to young men, in such style and manner that, had it not been for his pretended connection with Andover, he would have been repulsive. Now I happen to believe that no such individual as this Professor C. ever resided in Andover.

But I have not finished this chapter. Young men little know, and old men will scarcely believe when they are told of it, what an amount of human misery, under the forms of debility and disease, are inflicted upon children, by parental transgressions, of the kind to which these remarks refer; and so much might be said, without exhausting the subject, that I hardly know how or where to begin.

Thousands, perhaps I should say tens of thousands, are born every year in the United States, who, in consequence of venereal disease in those from whom, under God, they derive their existence, never enjoy health. They are sufferers greater or less, from the beginning of life to the very end of it. And not a few are so greatly diseased that they perish from the earth almost as soon as they are born into it.

Something like a quarter of a century ago, a case in point occurred in Charlestown, near Boston; of which I had some particular knowledge. It was that of a dissipated sea-captain, who, having become tired of a sea life, concluded to settle down, and make it his home on the land. He was already somewhat advanced in life; I think he was about fifty.

He married an excellent woman, much younger than himself, by whom he had several children. The first of these was shocking to behold. It was little more, at best, than a semi-putrid mass. It was not till after the birth and death of this child,—and these events came pretty near together,—that I knew in what a dreadful condition his system was, both the solids and the fluids.

The second child survived a considerable time, but was never healthy. It was as full of tubercles as if it had been for twenty years dying of consumption. Tenacious of life, exceedingly so, as the young are, it numbered some six or seven years before it perished; but it did not die till it had been a very great sufferer.

The third was healthier; it appeared to take the mother's constitution, at least in part. I believe it to be alive yet. It is, however, by no means vigorous; neither are two other living children, who were born subsequently. The eldest of the last two I have named is, however, one of those "shining marks" in which, it is said, death delights.

If it is better "to be," than "not to be," under the worst circumstances,— and some hold to this opinion — — then it is better, of course, that these three feeble children of a vicious and intemperate, and only half-reformed father should have had existence; even though they are "the poor inheritors of smart," by virtue of that law of God which renders it necessary that the sins of the parents should be visited upon children to the third and fourth generation, and, perhaps, to the thousandth.

How must such a father as this feel, unless his heart is adamant, to see his family falling around him one after another, while yet just entering on the threshold of existence!—and all because he could not deny himself the gratification of his appetites, even for a few short moments! Alas for human selfishness, and forbidden pleasures!

It may not be amiss to append to this chapter two cases which go farther to illustrate this part of our subject — derived from the pages of "The Boston Medical Journal," for May 3d, of the present year. They were communicated by a highly respected physician of Boston, and were of very recent occurrence.

The first case was comparatively a mild one. The child appeared to do well till it was about three months old. About this time the head and face became affected with "superficial ulcerations, most of them covered with crusts." Soon the symptoms became more severe. The child's head became "swollen and livid, and it was evidently on the verge of suffocation." On examination, "the nose was found completely plugged by some hard substance, which proved to be a mass of bone covered with inspissated mucus!" The physician had no doubt that the child had been congenitally affected, and treated it accordingly. At length it recovered; though not without such a loss of the bony parts of the interior of the nose, as seemed to depress considerably this organ, and give to the features for life a disagreeable expression.

In the second case, though the child was remarkably plump, at birth, and apparently healthy, yet it soon began to lose its appetite and its flesh till it became.

so puny that, at the age of two months, all hope of rearing it had been given up. "The skin," moreover, "was covered with a scaly eruption of a copper or brownish hue, most abundant about the nates, the limbs, and the face. The trunk did not present any spots. There was obstinate ulceration about the nail of one of the great toes, and the nail had been thrown off. Smaller ulcers and cracks existed about the anus and labia, and also upon the face." The father was an intemperate man; his other habits were not examined! The child died in a few weeks, after having been a terrible sufferer. There was no doubt with regard to the cause.

The mother of the child, moreover, had lost two children before, very suddenly, and under the influence of suspicious symptoms.

Most young men when they approach the end of their earthly career, especially if that career has been a dishonorable one, would gladly live their lives over again. Even Dr. Franklin expressed the desire to correct, in the second edition of his book, certain errors of the first.

A wise Providence has forbidden us this privilege; but has granted us another almost equal to it. A father's heart is bound up in his children, as Jacob's was in Joseph; and even in Joseph's children — his own grand-children. We take such an interest in children and grand-children, that we may be said, not unaptly, to live our lives over again in them. In the case of the Charlestown father, what is the hope?

When will men so live that these second editions of the book, as Franklin would call them, may, indeed, be more perfect than the first? Not, most surely, till our young men learn to revere God's holy and perfect laws; and the physical laws, no less than the moral ones.

CHAPTER VII.

THE PHYSICAL LAWS OF MARRIAGE.

I HAVE asserted and fearlessly maintained that every young person should look forward to marriage, at suitable age and under proper circumstances, as a moral duty. This opinion I cannot recall or alter. Entering, then, within the pale, as it were, of this institution, let us inquire concerning its laws.

Did fathers hold familiar conversation with their sons, and mothers with their daughters, on this important subject, and did the young make their parents their oracles instead of trusting to sources of information, which, at best, are very questionable, we should not find so many of both sexes rushing within the precincts of this sacred enclosure as ignorant of the first principles of matrimonial law as if no such law had ever existed.

Since the publication of the Young Man's Guide, — now nearly a quarter of a century ago, — I have received visits or letters, and sometimes both, from young men belonging to nearly every portion of this western world, and even to Europe. Among the number of my visitors and correspondents, have been some of our best educated young men — graduates, perhaps with honors, of Yale, Harvard, Amherst, etc.

One of these liberally educated young men came to me, a few years ago, at the close of a lecture on the physiology of marriage, at which he had been present, and taking me by the hand, with all that affection which he was wont to express towards his own father, not only thanked me for the information he had that evening received, but solicited farther instruction. He said that the thoughts to which he had been led, by the lecture, were not only new, many of them, but to him, as a recently married man, of the utmost importance.

It is not so, however, with all our liberally educated young men. Some few of them receive, it is true, a smattering of instruction on this topic, from the president or one of the professors under whom they have studied. But the far greater proportion of our students, both in colleges and elsewhere, care nothing at all about it, except so far as it gratifies a morbid curiosity.

I am, however, acquainted with one venerable president of a college in this country, who is, in this respect, as well as in a thousand others, like a father to his pupils. Nay, I even do him injustice in saying no more. Few fathers in the world act so truly the part of a father — I mean at this slippery period of life — as he.

But, if our liberally educated young men are, for the most part, not only exceedingly ignorant of the functions and laws of their bodies, but willing to remain so, how much worse must it be with the vast majority of the young, with their fewer and less favorable opportunities for information? Are they not almost as unfit to assume the semi-sacred responsibilities, so soon to devolve upon them in matrimonial life, as the beasts that perish?

It is but a very short time since one of the better sort of these uninformed young men joined me as I was walking along, with considerable luggage, towards a distant railroad depot, and begged the favor of carrying one of my parcels. He had attended my lectures and had read some of my writings; and was greatly anxious for a few moments conversation.

As we passed along, he very modestly and cautiously introduced several of the topics which are discussed in this book. He was amiable, sensible, and in many things well-informed; though not very familiar with books and school. As a sailor, he had traversed the world from the seventy-third degree of north to the sixtieth degree of south latitude; and not only knew something of human nature, generally, but — what is much more difficult — something of himself. He was, moreover, conscientious, and desirous to know the truth, in order that he might love and obey it. He was frank and confiding; and in great earnest.

Seldom if ever, have I met with a young man to whom I could hopefully impart more truth, in half an hour, than to him; and I left him with feelings of regret, and with a new interest in this class of my fellow-men. Can it be, I said — must it be so — that young men are left by their parents and friends in such deplorable ignorance? Something they know — the most ignorant of them — of business, and books, and politics, and religion; but what do they know of themselves? What do they know of the house they live in?

There are mysteries everywhere — it must be so, under a government which is administered by such a Governor as ours is — so much above us, in his perfections and attributes. But is there a greater mystery, anywhere, than this general ignorance on a subject which everybody knows to be of almost paramount importance?

The first question asked by inquiring young men, who are fairly within the matrimonial enclosure, usually is, "What is right, with regard to sexual intercourse?" "Here we are," say they, "with our appetites and passions urging us on; and yet we are fully assured there is a limit which we ought not to pass. Tell us, if you can, where that limit is."

But, in order to reply, in the best possible manner, to such a question as this, much time is required. Were I asked, by an individual, how much he ought to eat, or drink, or sleep, or how much clothing, or what kind of clothing he ought to use, by day or by night, I could tell him something at random immediately; but to tell him rationally and scientifically, could not be the work of a moment.

I must first know very particularly about his habits, hereditary and acquired; both as regards health and disease. I must know something also of his education, and of his temper and temperament. I must, in short, to do justice, either to him, or to myself, and the cause I serve, make a thorough physiological examination. It would be comparatively easy to lay down a code of abstract rules, without these preliminaries; but judiciously to adapt or apply them to his particular case and circumstances, would be the proper work of a much longer period. It would even be desirable to live by him, and to see him at various times, and under various circumstances.

Just so with the instructions to be given with reference to the physiology of marriage. Twenty years ago I asked a most excellent man, of great age, observation, and experience — one, moreover, whose praise was in "all the churches," what he should regard as matrimonial excess. He hesitated, at first. Much, he said, would depend on circumstances. What would be excess in one person of a certain temperament and of a particular age, would be but moderation in another — all of which to a certain extent, even to an extent much greater than that to which he would have carried it, is true. However, he concluded at length, that as a general rule, any thing beyond twice a week, for him and his companion, would be excess.

On relating this conversation, sometime afterward, (of course without giving names) to an experienced physician, he remarked, that as many indulgences as two in a week would destroy him and many others — persons even of average constitutions.

I have made extensive inquiry on this subject — of all sorts and conditions of men. One very aged New England clergyman — who had been the husband of four wives — told me that after fifty long years of observation, experience and reflection, he had come to the full conclusion that, for literary and sedentary men, however robust and healthy, any thing of this kind beyond once a month would partake of the character of excess; although he well knew that in some circumstances, and for a time, a much greater indulgence could not only be borne, but seemed, at first view, to be even beneficial.

Some of my readers may perhaps be already aware that the far-famed, and very far-hated, Sylvester Graham taught a doctrine not greatly unlike that of the preceding paragraph. A frequency of sexual indulgence greater than that of the weeks of the year, he said was absolutely inadmissible; while, as a general rule, it would be better for both sexes — no less than for posterity — if the indulgence were restricted to the number of lunar months.

This doctrine, it is true, so utterly at war with the general habits and feelings of mankind, was almost enough, at the time it was announced, to provoke the cry of, Crucify him. Indeed, I have often thought that while the public odium was ostensibly directed against his anti-fine flour and anti-flesh eating doctrines, it was his anti-sexual indulgence doctrines, in reality, which excited the public hatred and rendered his name a by-word and a reproach. But, as a belief in the great doctrine of the circulation of the blood, though it gained little credence, while Dr. Harvey, the discoverer, was alive, began to gain ground as soon as he was dead, so Mr. Graham was hardly dead, — and not at all entombed — ere the views which he proclaimed, on this subject began to find favor, both in this country and in Europe.

At the present time, I doubt whether there are a dozen men of sound science, in the ranks of physiology and hygiene, to be found in the known world, who will object to the soundness of Mr. Graham's views on this particular topic. They seem to discover, in the constitutional habits and tendencies of woman, what was the original intention and purpose of high Heaven, in a matter concerning which, specifically, revelation does not determine.

A few indeed have gone much farther, at least in theory. Assuming that the sole object of the sexual instinct and its apparatus, is the reproduction of the species, and that to this great end, exclusively, every "congress" should be directed, they would limit the recurrence of the act to the mutual desire of the parties to become parents.

But is there not room for doubt, after all, whether this was the whole of the Divine intention? For, if it were so, why should the power of procreation continue, in our sex, when not abused, as long, or nearly as long as life? And why should the susceptibility to pleasure, in the other sex, continue beyond the age to which child bearing is limited?

Is it not much more probable, all things and circumstances taken into the account, that, by the Divine plan, the gratification of the sexual instinct is determined, as Graham and others have thought, by the menstrual period, at least while that function continues? For, we must not forget, as one item in our estimates, that if woman, by virtue of her own constitutional tendencies, independent of mis-education or perversion, ever makes any advances towards the other sex, *as* a sex, except perhaps during pregnancy, it is soon after the cessation of the menstrual discharge. May we not, hence, infer that this function, while it prepares for the commerce of the sexes, at the same time limits its frequency?

On this point, however, I speak, as it becomes me, with some diffidence. For, I am by no means sure that our most ultra physiologists are not very near the truth, after all. I am by no means certain that Scripture revelation — to say nothing of physiology — in its most rigid interpretation, does not restrict us to the simple purpose of perpetuating the race. I am, however, quite sure that one indulgence to each lunar month, is all that the best health of the parties can possibly require.

It will be said, I know — it has often been so said — that if this is the law, it is a most rigid one. And so, indeed, at first view, it may seem. But what, then? Am I at fault, in announcing it? I certainly *did* not *make* the law. At most, I am but its interpreter. So far as I can see, and so far as close reasoning, both from analogy and the nature of the case, can carry me, it presents itself to my own mind as a most excellent law.

For, have we not already seen that the amount of human enjoyment to be derived from the appetites is not graduated by frequency of indulgence, so much as by infrequency? That it is not he, for example, who is almost always eating and drinking, who obtains, even for the time, the most gustatory enjoyment; but oftener the reverse? So, in my own view, with the sexual appetite.

If this last is indulged too frequently, although it might sometimes happen that the power to enjoy and the sum total of our enjoyment would increase for a time, yet both of them will prematurely fail. It is a general law that they who give themselves up to early and persevering indulgence, become early impotent, or at least lose, early, their susceptibility to venereal pleasures — and, indeed, to all sorts of pleasure — while they who are more self-denying, retain their powers and their pleasures to the end of life; or at least to a very late period.

It is, moreover, worthy of notice that the pleasures of love, no less than the strength of the orgasm, are enhanced by their infrequency. It is, in this also, as in eating and drinking. Eating twice or three times a day probably gives us more gustatory enjoyment than eating half a dozen or a dozen times during the same period. Nor does frequent eating sooner wear out or spoil the appetite than frequent sexual indulgence. It is by no means certain that the smallest number of meals a day which is compatible with health — I mean one, only — would not give, to any of us, who are adults, a greater quantity of gustatory enjoyment, taking the whole of life together, than a greater number. We certainly enjoy most when we have the most perfect appetite; but this perfect appetite we seldom have. Real hunger is usually anticipated. We seldom **wait** long enough for our food to be really hungry. In other words we eat before we are hungry, and hence are seldom if ever hungry.

From what we know of the ways and works of God, it is hardly a presumption to infer that strict conformity to his holy laws, physical not less than moral, will in the end, taking only this short and uncertain life into the account, give us the most of enjoyment. The heaven below does not conflict at all with the heaven above; but is part and parcel of the same thing.

If the maximum frequency of sexual commerce be the gradually recurring lunar months — if, I mean to say, this doctrine can be fairly inferred from a strict and honest interpretation of the Divine law — then it is to be presumed that in rigidly conforming to this arrangement we shall in the end secure the most pleasure, even if this little life were our all. It is probably so, I mean to say, as a general rule; to which however, as to most general rules, there may be more or fewer exceptions.

Or if this should not be admitted, it *must* be admitted that by carrying out God's plan to the full extent of the most rigid self-denial which his law really requires, we gain the most of happiness, physical, social, intellectual, and moral, on the whole and in the end. We shall be best satisfied with ourselves in the final review.

I have qualified these remarks by saying, "as a general rule." It was meet that I should do so. We are made, as a race, and normally, to last on to old age, and must govern our conduct in all the every-day concerns of life, on the presumption that we shall do so. Nevertheless we may be killed to-morrow at Norwalk; or drowned next week in some *Arctic*. On these last exigencies, however, we may not and should not calculate.

As an additional argument against the too frequent indulgence of the sexual propensity, and an argument, too, which is not without its weight, it should be observed that one of Europe's most able philosophers — the celebrated Montesquieu — is said to have been begotten on the evening of a re-union of his parents, after a separation of many long years.

But however this may be, in point of fact, we know one thing, that prostitutes seldom conceive; and still more rarely give birth to living, healthy children. Still further, we know how common it is, with the young, who give way to their feelings, *ad libitum*, in early married life, to remain a long time without any issue. These and numerous other considerations, taken together, certainly mean something; and should not, by the wise, be overlooked.

But young men, as we have seen, are usually without information; and hence seem to suppose that within the pale of matrimonial life there is no limit to indulgence except that which grows out of a due respect for woman — rather, I should perhaps say, to a good and faithful beast of burden — and some degree of regard to their own immediate suffering. Hence it is that the first months of matrimonial life are, so often, little better than a season of prostitution, except that it has not yet been stigmatized with the name. Hence, too, one reason why we have so many still born, prematurely born, and sickly children; as well as why we lose one half of all who are born under ten years of age.

A young man near the metropolis of New England, who had been married to a very active, healthy young woman less than a year, and, who, from being hale and robust at the time of marriage, had become pale, emaciated, cadaverous, feeble, and irresolute, seemed, at length, to be on the verge of a galloping consumption. It is quite possible that he might have inherited a tendency to this dread disease from his ancestors; for nothing, as we shall see hereafter, is more common than a connection between this tendency and undue amativeness. Of this however, in the case before us, I have no reliable information.

A young neighbor of his, who was a disciple of mine, and had read much on the subject, said to him famiiarly one day, "Sam, don't you know what ails you?" "No, I don't," said he, "except that, as the doctor says, my nerves are very weak." "Has the doctor told you nothing more?" "No." "Then I can tell you." So he proceeded, with great freedom, and frankness, and good humor, to bring home to his mind such charges that the wretched invalid made immediate confession to nine or ten months of daily indulgence. My young friend in the further exercise of his pity and benevolence, gave him the best counsels of which he was capable, and left him. Nor were his counsels unheeded. A new world was opened to the transgressor. In a year more he was nearly recovered; and he is still living and at the head of a small, though rather sickly family.

Some of the blinded devotees of sensuality may here inquire, and with much apparent shrewdness, — for Satan and his friends are seldom wanting in this commodity — whether it is not quite probable that this young invalid, during the nine or ten months aforesaid, secured to himself such an aggregate of enjoyment that he could afford to be still for a time. "Here were some two or three hundred indulgences," it may be said, "while the philosophy or physiology you advocate would hardly allow us more than two or three times this number in a whole life time."

In answering this inquiry and objection — by no means unfair after all — several things are to be considered. It should be understood that the young transgressor was rendered almost impotent at the time my young friend met with him and put him into the right path; and that his course, but for this timely interview, seems to have been almost run. Suppose, however, he had been left to go on to the last stages of consumption, and had died the next year or next but one; will it be claimed that with such an end before him, he acted the wise, or even the truly selfish part? Would this have been to secure the highest possible measure of amative enjoyment?

Suppose, however, that, though in his restoration to a measure of his former general health and vigor, his virile powers were never entirely regained, is it not possible — nay is it not *quite* probable — that he was thus actually a loser of at least one half of that sexual enjoyment, which God, in his providence, and in virtue of his original physical organization, had kindly designed for him?

But then again, admit that he did not seize and appropriate to his own use *quite* one half of all the physical sexual enjoyment God had provided for him as the inheritance of a life time, still was it no drawback or reduction from the remaining one half to remember that he had involved another, more dear to him, if possible, than himself, in a punishment, which though unlike his own, could scarcely, in the aggregate, be less in amount — and not her alone, but his children, too, should he ever have any?

Was it — would it have been — no draw-back upon the short-lived pleasures of sex, allotted to him, to be obliged, as the result, to consult or employ, a host of physicians attendants, or apothecaries, and to pay another host of bills of expense? Was it no draw-back upon the happiness of his after life to be obliged to watch, with fearful tremblings and forebodings, the issue of some scores of childrens' diseases — to say nothing of the performance of the last sad duties to the departed? Would it have been nothing to see his children, in the sequel of a long and painful sickness, go down, one after another, into the silent grave?

It is as utterly impossible that the young should escape these consequences of parental transgression — whether that transgression takes place within or without the precincts of matrimonial life — as to resist, effectually, the laws of attraction and gravitation. It is indeed true, as before admitted, that the evils of early abuse, before the age of twenty-five, are more numerous, and certain, and severe, than the others. The same law of hereditary descent prevails in both cases; and the same God reigns above, to visit iniquity by the appointed agencies, in his own time and manner.

It is proper to remark, however, that sexual indulgence, for some reason or another — both solitary and social — seems to be pursued, with more eagerness, by consumptive, nervous and delicate people than any other. It certainly is so within the pale of matrimonial life. It is curious, also, to observe, as I have said already, that it is persons of this very class or description who are soonest and most certainly injured or destroyed by it.

A young couple had been recently married, both of

whom had inherited a tendency to pulmonary consumption. It is true that they had not, till now, experienced any symptoms of the disease. Suddenly, however, I was called to visit them. They were going downward as fast as the wheels of time, and of sensuality, could carry them; especially the husband.

My prescription and counsels had sole reference to the removal of the cause of the diseased symptoms, and were apparently efficacious. An entire or almost entire non-intercourse law, in the progress of a year or two, gave them both, once more, a tolerable constitution, though by no means a strong one; and what is more, under Providence, gave them a family of comparatively healthy children. Nearly twenty years have elapsed, and they are still in the land of the living. Have not twenty years of moderation been worth more than one year of brutal excess would have been?

I have alluded to the opinion, quite common with the young of our sex, that marriage is, or may be, a state of unrestrained intercourse. So far is it from being the design of the great author of this institution, to render it a scene of unlicensed indulgence, or, in other words, of habitual, practical prostitution, that I have no doubt the intention was the reverse of all this. Instead of encouraging indulgence without limit, one of its very designs appears to me to teach us self-restraint and self-denial. Nor could the Divine Being give us, as far as I can see, a more favorable school for this purpose.

Man, to repeat what has been repeatedly affirmed,

already, is coarse and sensual — he needs to be polished and purified. Both of these offices, marriage, when rightly understood and properly regarded, never fails to accomplish. It does not require celibacy or the nunnery on the one hand, nor does it permit indulgence on the other. It simply requires us to be men and women; but it demands that we should be rational men and women, and not mere brutes. Above all, it does not permit us to be brutes of the lowest and most degraded cast. It seeks to reinstamp on us that Divine image which by disobedience we have lost.*

One eminent man among us is wont to say that it is in matrimonial life, and especially in those circumstances in which we are delegated with a kind of sub-creative power, that we approach nearer than in any other place below the sun to Jehovah's spotless throne.

Is it not passing strange, that with the Bible in his hands, any intelligent person should hold forth the doctrine that man, in the gratification of his various appetites, is a creature of mere instinct, on a level with the brutes? Yet such assertions have been heard. Be assured they are not in accordance with reason, revelation, or sound sense.

* I might make more of this idea, if space permitted. Paradoxical as it may seem, it is scarcely too much to say, that one of the very *ends* of marriage is gradually to purify us wholly from sensuality, by bringing our bodies under that law of which Paul makes so much in his writings.

CHAPTER VIII

A FUNDAMENTAL ERROR.

No one has a right to forget, either within the pale of matrimony or elsewhere, that by a general law as irrevocable as the laws given at Mount Sinai amid thunderings and lightnings — and emanating from the same Divine source — like begets its like. Not that the child always resembles, in every particular, the mother, or any one of the remoter relatives; indeed such a result is but seldom. Still a resemblance there will be, to some or all of them; and not unfrequently a resemblance, so striking, to some one of them that we speak of it, in terms not unlike the following:— "How much that child looks like its father!" or "That boy is the very picture of his mother!" or "James looks as much like his uncle Richard as if he were his own son!"

According to Alexander Walker and others who have made extensive observations on this subject, it often happens that when the general features — as indicated by the frame work of the face — and the vital organs resemble those of one parent or progenitor, the locomotive part, or the bony and muscular systems, resemble those of the other; and the contrary. So that when we say of a particular child, that it is the very picture of one or another of its relatives, we do not necessarily deny that in some things he may also resemble others. In truth, if the doctrines above mentioned are well founded, we rather affirm it.

Perhaps it is not too much to say, in plain English, that every child is and must be a combination of various qualities derived from the stock or breed; and that these qualities are in different proportions. Here, in one, there is more of the character, physically, of the mother; there, in another, of the father. And, in a few instances, we follow a remoter ancestor more closely than our own immediate parents.

Another circumstance greatly modifies human character. It is the condition of parents, as regards temper, health, and a thousand other things, at the time of conception. The child's character, though substantially built up on that of the whole ancestry as a basis — but resembling some one of that ancestry, more than any other — is yet, in no trifling degree that of the parents, at the moment above mentioned; especially of that parent, whom, in constitution he most follows.

Some have made too much of the last species of influence. They seem to have supposed that character, in after life, was almost wholly dependent on the parental state of body, mind and heart, at the moment whence we date our fœtal existence. But I am satisfied, most fully, that this is carrying the matter quite too far.

David says, in one of his Psalms: — "Behold I was shapen in iniquity, and in sin did my mother conceive me." I do not suppose, however, that in thus pouring out, as it were, his very soul, and bemoaning, before God, his sinfulness, David intended to express the exact physiological truth. His language, doubtless, partakes largely of the figurative, like that of the orientals generally. And yet it may have been, in part, true, physiologically. The best of us are greatly shaped in guilt and sin, unless descended from a race that has never apostatized. Nor is it too much to say that the best of us transmit the effects of guilt and sin to those who come after us, down to the third and fourth, if not to the three hundredth and four hundredth generations.

The condition of David, as indicated by the most literal interpretation of his language is, almost without exception, the condition of our race. We are conceived, generally, under many unfavorable circumstances; and some of us under the worst circumstances possible. But this broad statement will be better understood and more likely to be received, when it is accompanied by a few explanations.

Each day of our existence is, as it were, a little life. From the death of sleep we are raised every morning — and by nothing less than Almighty Power — to a new and wonderful existence. But we are not raised to our wonted full strength and perfection at once. There are stages or gradations of each daily or miniature life, as well as of the life that is measured out by threescore years and ten.

Rest and sleep do, it is true, partly restore us, but not wholly. This may be seen by comparing the state of the pulse at rising, with its condition at nine or ten o'clock of the forenoon; as well as by many of the other functions of the body. The pulse, though quicker, is not so full and strong in the morning, as it is about the middle of the forenoon. When we have been abroad, more or less, and inhaled more or less the pure air and drank in the pure light of Heaven, and used more or less all our powers of body, mind, and spirit, the motion of the heart, arteries, lungs, brain, etc., though it may be slower, becomes at the same time stronger; and we rise to what might, perhaps, be called the flood-tide of the human system.

This highest, most perfect state of humanity, physically speaking, this flood-tide of the vital and sanguineous circulation takes place, as already intimated, at about nine or ten o'clock. It varies, however, with our varying state of health or debility, with the earliness or lateness of our rising, with the state of our stomach, our mental apparatus, our affections, and many more circumstances.

At this summit, this very highest pinnacle of our existence — this physical Pisgah of humanity — we are best prepared to survey the land before us, and go forth to its possession. For devotion, study, labor, amusement, conversation, and even for the gratification of our appetites, we are best prepared, and probably best disposed. And other things and circumstances being equal, I cannot help thinking that in propagating ourselves at this highest point of human elevation, we should best accomplish, in one respect at least, our earthly mission.

It is indeed true that everything cannot be done at once. If the early morning hours must be given to devotion and study — as seems perhaps most natural — it is obvious that eating, drinking, amusement, labor, etc. must wait. Or if, as with many — perhaps the most of our people in civilized life — the gratification of the stomach, and daily labors, and amusements occupy the first place, then devotion and study must either be deferred for a time or hurried, or otherwise so conducted as to be greatly diminished in value.

I do not mean to affirm that the varied duties of human life, with its pleasures, too, cannot be performed, by the robust and healthy, at almost any part or hour of the day, or even of the night, should circumstances require it; for they certainly can be. But they can be most worthily performed, no doubt, when we are, so to speak, most truly alive; that is, when we are nearest to the top of our condition.

As we pass from nine or ten to twelve or one o'clock, in the progress of our daily journey, our strength of body and mind — for these must accompany each other — gradually decline; as is shown by a quicker, more frequent, and consequently more feeble pulse, as well as by a more excitable but less energetic state of the cerebral and nervous systems. Refreshment and rest, from time to time, of suitable quality and quantity, may somewhat retard the ebbing tide; but the check, after all, will be temporary. The waters will recede, gradually, till evening — in general till we retire for rest — when it will be ebb-tide.

If we sit up unusually late, we are not only at ordinary low water mark, but very low — so low that our usual hours of sleep do not always restore us. We are, in a measure, diseased. Our nerves are over excited; our arterial and respiratory movements are accelerated; and our organs of sense become in some respects clamorous. I do not mean to affirm that our sensual powers — our appetites — are strengthened at this time; for it is the reverse. They are weakened in just proportion to their increased activity and demand, etc., for gratification. If nuts, cider, cakes, oysters, eggs, ice creams, music and other indulgences are demanded, it is a morbid or diseased demand, and not a natural or healthy one. "Tired nature's sweet restorer, balmy sleep," is the only gratification which the healthy system can require or demand, at nine, ten or twelve o'clock at night.

In short, the human being, at the hour of ordinary retirement to rest, is in a febrile state. This miniature fever is indeed more perceptible in the case of the feeble, the over-fatigued, or the over-indulged; and of those who, as I said before, sit up very late; but it exists in all. Happy is it, when it is not carried to a degree that exposes us to danger from acute or severe disease — fever, croup, palsy, apoplexy, etc.

Thousands of our race perish, not at the height of this daily fever, but during its decline, or near what might be called its termination. They perish, in one word, during what medical men would call the collapse, which follows the previous excitement. They have labored, or studied, or amused themselves all day, and perhaps during a long evening besides; and to late hours and a febrile state they have added new indulgences, if not new excesses. Perhaps they have spent their evening at a concert, a ball, or a levee, till it is eleven, twelve, or one o'clock. At two, or three, or four, the fever subsides, and nature yields, in collapse. The vital powers, *depressed* and *oppressed*, are unable to rally; nature struggles a short time, but ineffectually; the curtain falls, and the scene closes.*

This is, briefly the history of a very considerable portion of our transgressing race, especially in this land of abundance and of freedom to indulge our

* Since the above was written I have seen an article copied from the "Foreign Quarterly" into the "National Magazine," which confirms the statements I have here made, in a most striking manner. The writer in the Quarterly says he deduced his conclusions from observations on 2,880 deaths of persons of all ages; and his conclusion is in these words: — "The least mortality is during the mid-day hours, viz, from ten to three o'clock; the greatest, during early morning hours, from three to six o'clock." The maximum of deaths, he says, is from five to six o'clock in the morning.

appetites. The subject is more painful in the review, from the consideration that so many of our ablest citizens, particularly our statesmen, judges and other public officers, have perished in this way; and what is truly a little remarkable, not a few of them at a particular hour of the night, or rather at an early hour of the morning, and at the climacterical period of sixty-three.

In most persons, of course, at least for a considerable time, say for twenty, forty, or sixty years, the current of life, conjoined with the force of long habit, is so strong, even in the collapse of which I have spoken, as to carry them by the point of danger; and hence they continue to live on. It is, however, to the physiologist a matter of no little surprise that they *should* do so.

But I have made these preliminary and preparatory remarks, in part, that you may be in readiness for the doctrine announced by the Shepherd-King of Israel; and, in part also, to show you, by physiological reasoning, their bearing and correctness in their application to the human race generally. I wished to show you how it is that, as a race, — whatever David may or may not have intended, and whatever may have been the facts in relation to him, — we are all conceived in sin, and shapen in iniquity.

It is, however, hardly necessary that I should state to an American reader the palpable and indisputable fact that it is precisely from the hour when nature, all exhausted, depressed and feverish, — not to say when she is suffering under a load of abuse, — sinks, collapses and is, as it were, almost ready to "beat a retreat," that we date, as individuals, our existence. It is when we are nearest the point where we are fit for nothing but "tired nature's sweet restorer," that we perform one of the most responsible, I had almost said, most serious duties devolving upon humanity.

Suppose it could be true,— what some of our phrenologists, and perhaps a few of our physiologists, have told us, that, as is the parent physically and morally at the important moment of conception, so is the child, — how long would it take to extinguish utterly, the vital flame which God has breathed out upon the earth in which we have our abode? How many centuries could pass before man, made at first in the image of God, would absolutely become extinct?

But we may be assured that, though greatly abused and crippled in a thousand ways, we are not left, as a race, with the power of self-destruction so immediate and so inevitable. Deterioration there must, indeed, be in the matter of which we are now treating; deterioration there has indeed been, but there are redeeming circumstances, and let us be grateful to Almighty God that there are.

Still, the race to which we belong can never rise — we can never eject from this part of Jehovah's vast domain, "disease, and all our woe"— till a great and important change is effected in our habits. What that change must be, in all its phases, cannot be told in a single volume; nevertheless, I must, in this work, small as it is, point to first principles, and, at least, *suggest* the true means of laying broadly, and deeply, and firmly, a sure foundation.

One thing appears to me plain, that, if our race will continue to date their existence, physiologically and fœtally, at the most unfavorable and unfortunate hour of the whole twenty-four, we must remove all factitious things and circumstances. We must not render the human inheritance, physical, mental, or moral, worse than the direst necessity compels. Physically, intellectually, socially and morally, we must be at this sub-creative hour, — I had nearly said this most sacred of all hours, — in our approach to that marriage-bed, which an apostle has declared to be intrinsically " honorable," in as good a condition as the nature of the case will possibly admit.

It is often believed by the vulgar, and I am inclined to think not wholly without truth, that idiocy, partial or complete, has sometimes been the result of sexual commerce when under the influence of intoxication. It is even supposed that, to this end, it is not indispensable that both parents should be " inebriate," but only one. Now it would seem quite enough that humanity should be conceived when nature is at ebb-tide merely, without the addition of other deteriorating influences; and that this circumstance alone is sufficient to account for that physical deterioration of the race which is, everywhere in civic life, so obvious. One, I say, might come to this conclusion, without being very deep in the knowledge of physiology **or** hygiene. But when, in addition to all this, the parent's brain, during the day, has been steeped, as it were, in rum, tobacco, cider, wine, ale, tea, and coffee, particularly the former two, what has poor human nature to hope for?

Moreover, for every idiot, or half-idiot, formed by these larger abuses, conjoined with the general irritability and feverishness of the rundown and wornout machine, we have probably some scores, if not some hundreds, of quarter-idiots, so to call them; and some thousands, or ten thousands, whose intellects, if not their spiritual powers, are more or less affected and deteriorated, all the way from one fourth to one hundredth or one thousandth. For there are degrees of abuse in all the proportions herein indicated; and why should not the inheritance be in proportion to the abuse? Most certainly it is so.

The man who, without coming to the still evening hour half or one fourth intoxicated, is yet heated in his blood, and indeed throughout his whole system, by more or less of alcoholic drink, should not complain, of God or man, if he has sickly, imbecile or effeminate children. He is but reaping,— such is the law under which we live,— according as, in his folly, he has sown.

It is not distilled and fermented drinks alone, however, nor even these and tobacco, that pave the downward road, to which I am now endeavoring to direct the public mind, in order that there may be a timely escape. It is anything and every thing that, by excess in quantity or error in quality, poisons the vital current, or embarrasses the functions of the body or the mind. Every thing which is wrong in our food and drink; all unnecessary medication; and all cabins of bad air, from the counting-room or school-room of ten or twelve feet square, to the unventilated mechanic's shop or cotton factory of even gigantic dimensions, are as certainly doing us mischief during the day, as that two and two, when added together, make four; and are as certainly, though it may be not so rapidly, unfitting us for matrimony, physiologically considered, as rum and tobacco.

And then, again, it is not those things alone which affect the body and derange its mechanism; the mind, too, has its influence. He who, during the day, or any considerable part of it, has been the slave or the victim of anger, fear, grief, envy, melancholy, hatred, revenge, or even over anxiety, has been as certainly unfitting himself for the high prerogative of Paul's honorable marriage-bed, as if he had been under the influence of downright intoxication, only not in the same degree. How poorly fitted must the progeny of such circumstances be to form a meet temple for the indwelling of the Divine Spirit!

When I think what temperance, health, and general purity are required, not merely on occasions, but habitually, in order to become a parent, I can scarcely forbear to tremble. Is it not enough that we are willing to replenish the world from the very dregs, as it were, of life — the mere remnant of a worn out day, the cuttings and clippings of an old garment — but must we add to it the abuses of gluttony, intemperance, and perverted, and degrading, and depressing passions?

This suggests to every one who will but take the trouble to think at all, his whole duty in relation to this matter. He who aspires to the great work of increasing and multiplying and replenishing the earth, according to the directions given to the *first* Adam, must enter into the spirit and temper of the *second*. He must cultivate and elevate, were it only with reference to the improvement of his own progeny, his whole nature. He must, with a view to this important end, obey all the known laws of God, physical, intellectual, social and moral. He must elevate himself, aided by the Divine influences, to such a height of physical and moral excellence as may render him worthy of co-operating with the world's Master Spirit in the great work of human redemption.

You will have observed before now, that I do not say with much positiveness what definite course should be taken under the circumstances to which I have, in this chapter, called your attention. I have pointed to a fundamental error embodying, as it were, all our other errors; but have left it, thus far, to the good sense of my readers to apply the proper remedy. I must, however, in closing, endeavor to secure your attention to the subject a few moments more, by way of review.

Suppose you have in your family a drivelling idiot. To support him by your hard earnings might be borne, and borne easily; especially if you had no lurking suspicion or secret misgivings with reference to the part you had acted, in connection. But to bear with his weakness and folly; to be subjected day after day, and year after year, to all the physical, intellectual, moral, and social trials to which his condition must inevitably subject you — to the pain of thinking that, in all probability, you have been the cause of your and his suffering — how could your heart endure it?

Suppose, even, a state of things short of downright idiocy. Owing to your ill-health, or to other circumstances, you knew you were not in a proper condition to become the progenitor of a child. Yet, for the sake of a momentary gratification, and stimulated by external and internal heat, you incurred the risk. And now the iniquity of the father has been visited upon the child. He is weak, wayward, froward; in one word, hard to govern, as the phrase is. He is your child, and yet you are almost ashamed of him. He is to be educated; but you hardly know how. He has an immortal spirit, yet he has not character enough to encourage the hope of making on him any lasting good impressions. Alas! what trials may be in reserve for transgression, which timely light and truth may now prevent!

And then the slighter degrees of transgression have

their influence in forming fallen character; we hardly realize how much; nor shall we, in all probability, understand this matter as it truly is, till the last day shall reveal it. Our duty, however, so far as known, can be heeded. We can do what we already know to be right.

CHAPTER IX.

THE LAW OF PREGNANCY.

It is, to say the least, quite doubtful whether, on any point connected with the physiology of matrimony, young men from the ordinary walks of life are shrouded in thicker darkness than in regard to the laws of human gestation or pregnancy; and, if light is needed any where, is it not here?

On this subject, if on nothing else, I speak that to which, in the Providence of God, my attention has been so long and so extensively called that I may justly consider myself competent to testify. Young men, I say again, are in utter ignorance, or almost so, with regard to the laws of pregnancy. But then there is one redeeming thing about it, many are anxious to know them. This, so far, is encouraging. To find young men in the spirit of progression gives us hope. But to keep such young men no longer in suspense, let us proceed to our inquiry.

The savages of the wilderness, in some instances, as we are told, practise what might be called non-intercourse during the whole period of utero-gestation. This, if true, and I suppose it to be so, is a most remarkable, and, at the same time, most interesting fact in the history of mankind.

Some of the British and American physiologists, in pursuance of their investigations, have come to the conclusion that the savage state, in this particular instance, is the true state of nature. Surprising is it that it should be so. We have seen that our appetites are *fallen* appetites; now, can the appetites of the most degraded of our race be less fallen than those of the most elevated and cultivated?

Let us examine this matter,— for it will richly repay the trouble. Let us see, if we can, what the truth is; this precious commodity is sometimes found midway between extremes. In the present case the extremes of social life, refinement and barbarism, seem to meet, and to unite, in proclaiming entire abstinence during a long period of matrimonial life; while the general practice of the world of mankind proclaims, as we have elsewhere seen, an almost unlimited and unrestrained indulgence.

We will look at the subject, first, in the light of analogy; secondly, in that of anatomy, physiology, and hygiene; and lastly, in that of Christian morality.

For the purpose of deriving an argument from analogy, we will suppose the case of an intelligent young man who intends to keep pace with the spirit of the times. He sets out trees in his field or garden, or by the road-side, for usefulness, for shade, and for ornament; will he not take care of them from day to day, and from week to week? Will he not fence, water, and watch them, as he sees them need it? Most certainly he will.

Indeed, I know many a gardener and farmer, each of whose trees cost him, in various ways, a dollar or more a year. He protects them by boards or by stakes from external violence, as much and as well as he can. He knows full well that all hacking, bruising, galling, and peeling them would be greatly injurious. Accordingly he visits them from day to day, and even yearns over them with a degree of that tenderness with which a mother yearns over her offspring.

Other cares are needed. Perhaps the trees require watering and mulching in times of drought and heat. Perhaps there is need, at the approach of winter, of protecting them from the severe frost. His mind is ever and anon directed to the supply of their wants; and when he finds any one of them suffering or perishing, or even not making that progress which he had expected, he is grieved. In our intercourse with human beings we love most those whom we have most watched over and cared for, and suffered for; and hence, no doubt, one prominent source of parental love. And is it not true that, in conformity with this general principle, we become, in greater or less degree, attached to those plants, trees, and flowers, which we have watched over long and carefully?

Now what would be thought of him who should take exactly the opposite course to that which has just been suggested? What would be thought of the farmer or gardener, who, after digging a suitable number of holes in the ground, just about large enough to set posts in, and hastily crowding the expanding roots of a parcel of young trees into them and covering them, should leave them to themselves for months and years? No man who should do this could expect to retain, long, the reputation of a man of sense or skill in his profession. He could hardly retain a suitable degree of self-respect.

But if these things are so — if mere negligence would be disgraceful and disreputable — what would be thought of downright violence, or even of rough handling and treatment? What would be thought of him who should willingly, or by intention, disturb the roots of his young trees and shrubs, by the plough, the hoe, the spade, or the harrow, or in any other way; or who should recklessly wound, bruise, maim, or in any way disfigure them? If it is not workmanlike to neglect them, how much worse is it to agitate, enfeeble, or in any way, disturb them by the rude attacks of man or beast!

The same general remarks are applicable to planting and sowing; and with even more of force. Who is there that does not endeavor to leave the ground into which he has cast his seeds, in perfect quiet, during the first days, weeks and months, in order that the processes of germination and growth may have their perfect work? Who is he that would shake roughly, or in any way agitate the soil in which the young embryo plant was forcing its way into life? None, most certainly, but one who was entirely unfit for his business — an ignoramus, an idiot or a madman.

Again, in the management of domestic animals of all sorts; who is he that wholly neglects the well-being of the young in embryo? Above all, who is he — where is he to be found — who not only neglects but exposes it, willingly, to violence? We are bound, always, to be merciful to our beasts, as Solomon has intimated; but some men do not come up to Solomon's standard in ordinary every day circumstances. Many an individual treats his domestic animals with great roughness, from time to time — not to say with much of cruelty. Yet where is the individual to be found who will treat his animals, with young, with violence and cruelty? It would be to act in opposition to his own interest. If cruelty and violence were ever justifiable — and would ever comport with good policy — it would not be in circumstances like these.

We will now apply our remarks to the young of the human race, and thus finish our analogy. If sound sense and good policy — to say nothing of mercy — would lead us to do all in our power for the nutrition and development in the best and healthiest and most approved manner, of our plants and animals, should we do less for our own offspring — those who are, as it were, a part of us — who are bone of our bone and flesh of our flesh? Will we, above all, with open eyes, and full assent, inflict violence of any kind on the young being in embryo? Or if a young man were reckless enough, of himself, to do this, would he not spare the companion of his bosom the pangs which his recklessness might inflict on her, at least if she were intelligent enough to know that the fœtus is susceptible of being affected by violence?

Yet such reckless young men there have been — such, I fear, there still are. They well know that as the plant or tree depends on the quiet, proper arrangement, moisture, strength of soil, etc., in which it grows, so the infant in the uterus is best sustained and perfected, when the mother's solids and fluids — as a soil in which it is placed — are in the best possible condition; and the roots, so to call them, of the little being, are most undisturbed by any species of violence. And yet knowing the fact, they practically disregard it.

Thus far, the arguments to be derived from analogy, in their bearing on the case before us, are obviously in favor of non-intercourse during the whole period of utero-gestation. There is one more analogy remaining. It is mentioned last, not because it is regarded as of second or third rate importance, but because it is of such a nature as to render it very closely allied to our anatomical and physiological division. It is, in truth, — to give it the most appropriate name — a *fact*, derived from and based upon comparative physiology.

It has always struck me, as not a little remarkable that, in the providence of God, the whole animal world, below man, are restricted to non-intercourse, by their instincts. By the removal of the sexual instinct, during the long period of many months — in some instances, no less than nine — the process of uterogestation is wholly uninterrupted; and as appears most probable, not to say certain, the deterioration, no less than the destruction of the race, thereby prevented.

Now this arrangement of High Heaven, is either in accordance with Infinite Wisdom and Benevolence, and hence conducive to the highest good of the various tribes of animals, or it is not. Would we dare to say that it is not so?

But if non-intercourse, during pregnancy, is the law of Jehovah to all the tribes of animals below man, by what mode of reasoning shall it be made to appear that the law which is perfect for the brute, in a matter like this, is not perfect for man? True it is that we cannot always reason from brutes to men — so wide is the gulf between the two, at least when morally and religiously considered — but in the case before us, such reasoning appears to me legitimate. Heaven has thus made sure the perpetuity of the mere animal — without liability to deterioration — by an almost impassable barrier; while it has delegated to free agency, here, as well as elsewhere, the power "to counteract its own most gracious ends," if it chooses to do so.

There is another point to be considered; and here our comparison falls a little short. We are to remember that while in our dealings with the world of vegetation, the seed which produces a plant or tree is first separated entirely from the parent, and then cast out into a foreign soil, it is entirely different in the animal world. The young human tree, so to call it, is for many long months, on the parent tree; and only thrives as the parent thrives. It suffers also, if the parent suffers. In the formation of the fruit of a tree from the blossom, and in its preparation to be cast off or isolated from the parent, there may be a slight resemblance to those changes in the animal world which we are considering — but not so much in the germination and growth of the young shoot.

Now while the seed, in its germination, and the young shoot, in its growth, are, by their isolation, secured, on the one hand from all dangers which might be received through the parent, they are equally secured, on the other, from a necessity of that watch-care which is bestowed on the young animal, especially the rational one. The parent tree, of course, has no sense of responsibility for the right germination and growth of its progeny; and the parent of the mere animal is almost equally irresponsible, though in some respects, equally influential. But here, in the last instance, instinct is invoked; and to instinct the whole matter is assigned. In the case of the human animal, on the contrary, a most fearful responsibility is incurred.

There are a thousand things that have to do with the actual condition of the embryo human being, which are entirely within the control of the parents, but which are intimately connected with the well being of the child. Especially is it so when we look at the subject in the light of the laws of Anatomy and

Physiology, to some of the more important of which, I must now call your attention.

No one at the present day, can be wholly ignorant of the fact that a considerable proportion of the children born among us are still-born. So far as I have examined — and my opportunities for examination have not been confined to the crowded city, by any means — the proportion is about one in fifteen of all who are born. The proportion, moreover, appears to be increasing. But even at the present rate our annual national loss, from this source alone, can hardly be less than forty thousand.

This item of human mortality is believed to be, for the most part, the result of violence. All disease is indeed, in a general sense of the term, violence. But we mean something more than this, in the case of still-born children. They are, for the most part, destroyed by violence in the common, rather than the physiological and pathological acceptation of the term.

There are, indeed, numerous forms of violence to which the child in the uterus may be subjected. Among these are blows on the abdomen, externally; falls; violent efforts in amusement and labor; and great mental agitation, as by fear or grief. How these mental causes may have the effect of violence, so as to produce fœtal death, it may not be easy to say, in few words; and perhaps, in this particular instance you may as well assent to mere authority. But of all the forms of violence which are wont to inflict injury in the present case, none are so common as that violence to the whole nervous system which is produced during the terminus of sexual intercourse.

One of our most distinguished medical men — one who presumes to be a leader in the corps of his profession — is wont to say, with reference to still-born children, that they are killed by mechanical violence. His language on the subject is that of indignation; and will not, here, be repeated. It is just in its application, but it is severe; and approximates to the vindictive of the vulgar. The common sense of the mass of mankind — unenlightened as it now is — inclines in the same direction. Mechanical violence is better understood — is more tangible — than any other.

Without assuming that what everybody says must be true, it is nevertheless undeniable that this opinion has truth in it. There are brutes in human shape, of both sexes. There are those, especially of our own sex, who would not deny themselves one iota of immediate enjoyment, for the sake of joys remote, though ever so much magnified, if by so doing they knew they could save a wife from much future suffering, and an embryo child from certain destruction. Worse than even this. There are those of both sexes, as we shall see by and by, who would prefer the destruction of the child, and would choose violence of this very kind — if other forms were to fail — for its accomplishment.

But this is not the usual way in which children in the uterus are killed by violence. Scientific men are accustomed to explain the matter more in accordance with the laws of health and disease, as well as with analogies, such as have just now been presented.

They know, full well, that the embryo child thrives when the mother thrives. Give to her the most perfect health, in an uninterrupted stream, and the child can neither sicken and die, nor fail to be developed in due proportion and harmony. But take away from the mother any measure of this high and as some call it, perfect health,* and we take away in similar proportion, from the health and vigor of the child.

This healthful and vigorous state of the mother is always abated somewhat — I mean of course during gestation or pregnancy — by sexual indulgence. It is so, even if the mother takes little or no active part in it; but it is especially so when the contrary is the fact. The nervous orgasm is too great for the young germ. As certain processes of agriculture or horticulture, when carried on amid the newly set or recently germinated plants loosen their hold on the mother earth and cause them gradually to sicken, droop, and die, so does that agitation of the human being, to which I refer; especially when oft and frequently repeated.

Let me be understood, here. It is not affirmed that.

---

* Perfect health I suppose to mean, in general, immunity from fear and suffering — a sort of medium health, which passes for perfection. Such a thing as perfect health, in the physiological sense of the term, is not known to the present fallen world.

no mechanical violence is committed, to hasten on a fatal result, especially when the orgasm, both on the maternal and paternal side is strong; but only that it is, comparatively, inconsiderable in its effects. It is seldom, if ever, sufficient to produce the immediate destruction of the fœtus. The mischief comes in another way and manner.

First, the mother is herself weakened, through the attack on her nervous system; and whatever weakens her, even temporarily, weakens her offspring in utero. But, secondly, the child, dependent as it is upon the parent, is, in these circumstances, fed from a current of blood less rich and nutritive than it otherwise would be. The starvation system will do for adults much better than it will for the young in embryo.

Here, too, I greatly desire not to be misunderstood. One transgression of a healthy robust father or mother does not always kill, of course. Perhaps it may even seem to do no injury. Farther than this, even, may be true. Such persons may repeat the transgression to an extent that can only be measured by the term *frequently;* and yet the child may not be still-born. Healthy parents do not generally have still-born children as the result of this particular form of violence.

It does not hence follow that no injury is inflicted. The child in utero may be injured, doubtless often is so, without being destroyed; and the aggregate, or sum total, of these smaller inflictions may greatly exceed the mischief which is designated when we speak of a yearly loss of forty thousand children in the United States.

Children may come into the world with disease for their inheritance. They may be of a feeble and delicate organization. They may be feeble or erratic, mentally or morally. There is, indeed, no doubt that they often are so. I have seen parents of this description, who, out of a large family, had not a single healthy child. Every body wondered, and every cause was invoked, of the strange phenomenon, except the right — the frequent violation of the irrevocable laws of Heaven.

Of course I do not say that families may not be found of the description given in the last paragraph, where the cause of the debility or disease may be entirely different. The world abounds with causes of disease, both moral and physical. God works by means in this, as well as in other departments of his kingdom.

But if the children of very strong and healthy parents are more or less demented or diseased by sexual commerce during pregnancy; if there is always a tendency, even in the case of the robust, to the extinction of the child's vital energies, how much more is this the fact in the case of the great majority, whose physical inheritance is less favorable?

The whole truth should be proclaimed. Sexual intercourse during pregnancy, as a general rule, robs the child in the uterus, reduces its constitutional vigor, and predisposes it to various debilitating diseases; and, in some instances, as we have seen, quite extinguishes the flame of life. If forty thousand are killed outright every year, in the United States, in the uterus, it can hardly be doubted that some hundreds of thousands are *partly* killed. They are at least duly prepared to become the victims, sooner or later, of actual, it may be very severe, disease. Their minds, as well as their bodies, are somewhat deteriorated, especially in their tone or energy.

Now our young men — our old ones, too — should think of such facts as these whenever and wherever temptation solicits. Or if it should be said that they have not known the law, and hence know very little about the penalties annexed to its transgressions, then the proper reply is — they ought to know it. No young man who reads this book, and reads it through, shall be able to make the plea of honest ignorance hereafter. If I do not succeed in enlightening him, I will at least pioneer the way to truth and light. He shall know, at least, that there is something which he does *not* know.

I do not say that these considerations, standing by themselves, should compel us to the sweeping conclusion that all commerce of the sexes during gestation should be avoided; but they certainly point in that direction. They are to be taken into the account in settling the great question, and are entitled to weight.

Woman is also liable during pregnancy to abortion. This liability exists at every age, from puberty to the cessation of the menses. It is, however, on some accounts, a greater evil in proportion as it occurs early in matrimonial life; because, if it does not inflict a greater amount of immediate injury, it does, at least, render a person more liable to a recurrence of the same difficulty;—but it not unfrequently cripples her for life.

This abortion I say, then, even under the most favorable circumstances, is an evil. For its existence, as for still-births, there are many and various causes. Indeed, the same causes sometimes produce still-births and abortion both. But the most common cause is sexual indulgence, especially when it occurs at certain months of pregnancy.

It is most frequent during the first, toward the end of the third, and during the fourth month; and, also, about the seventh; but it may happen at any time during pregnancy, earlier or later. Against danger from this quarter, the female should be always strictly guarded; but especially so during the most dangerous seasons. She should even be aided by man in the work of guarding herself, as one of the highest of his offices. For woman alone, unaided, is not sufficient for this great work. What can she do without the co-operation of man? What, above all, can she do when man becomes her seducer? He is bound, as we have seen in an early chapter, by the special arrangement of Jehovah himself, to be her keeper. Does he perform, conscientiously, his duty?

Let him, henceforth, fully understand that **anatomy**

and physiology point to sexual commerce, during pregnancy, as one prolific source not only of still-births and abortion, but also of that whole train of smaller evils, which marshal themselves under these two leaders. Millions and millions of our race are slowly murdered in this way; while other millions, nay, other hundreds of millions,* are partly destroyed. And the destruction, in every degree, alights upon the soul as well as the body.

My most deliberate conviction is that if young men as a general rule, could see, at a single clear view, as they may perhaps see it in the review of the Great Day, all the diseases of mind and body to which, by their sensual indulgence during pregnancy, they subject their wives and children, they would hesitate in their career of thoughtlessness and recklessness They could not, with open eyes, bring mourning, la mentation and woe into their own houses, and to their own firesides and bed-chambers. They would govern themselves far better than now They would not, so often at least, prepare for themselves a world of misery before the time! They would wait a little! For, selfish as the world is, the number of young men who are so selfish as to be happy while they know they are the authors of suffering to their wives and children, must be very small indeed. The direct torment inflicted on themselves by a consciousness of such wrong doing, would be sufficiently dreadful; but this would not

* It is about fifty millions, as nearly as can be ascertained, to each generation of thirty years.

diminish the intensity of the suffering of others. It would still be immense and appalling.

There is one more form of suffering to the race, to which I have not yet adverted in particular. Thousands of fathers and mothers go far enough in transgression to cause premature labor, and a somewhat delicate offspring, while it can hardly be said that the general health of the child, or even of the mother, is seriously impaired by it. Still, it inflicts injury more or less, and should be avoided.

In the closing part of the volume, as well as in other parts of the work, I shall give such directions with regard to physical education prospectively, as the nature of the case demands.

This is the place to speak of sexual indulgence during pregnancy, as viewed in the light of Christianity. On this part of our subject I must be as brief as possible.

We should not forget that man is made, that is, designed, in the image of God. It is our duty, as Christians, to preserve that image. Nay, more; it is our duty to restore it as fast as possible, whenever and wherever it is lost. These remarks, I confess, amount to little more than the most common truisms. And yet, can it be that their force is duly apprehended when brought to bear upon the case before us?

It would seem to be a smaller detraction from the image of God to give a wrong direction to the plants and vines which we cultivate; or even to neglect to give them a *right* direction, than to give a wrong direction to the human being. God has, as it were, enstamped himself even on these; will we not do all we can to aid them in retaining his Divine image?

But if so; if not to give them a proper direction from the first were a species of wrong, is there nothing blameworthy in detracting from their value, or marring in them that structural perfection and beauty which reflect the character of their Author, and, in a sense, constitute his image? Does not he who recklessly loosens their roots, poisons them through their sap vessels, or withholds from them that nurture which he knows their advancing nature demands, — for every plant and tree must have its appropriate food, — detract from the image of a holy God, and a most kind and benevolent Father?

And then, too, by parity of reasoning, is there no guilt attached to a more direct, and I fear more general detraction from God's image, in marring and defacing and destroying that symmetry, beauty, health, mental force and moral worth, which, but for our interference might have been an instrument in blessing, in countless ways, this dark world? But all this, and much more than can be readily portrayed in a few short paragraphs is done every day, and in a thousand, if not ten thousand instances. He who begets a child in his own image, when that image is defaced by sin and guilt in any of their forms, is of that description. So is he who, by yielding to his lusts, at the expense of a child in embryo, prefers present pleasure to the future physical, intellectual, and moral happiness of his own offspring.

As I have frequently adverted to the effects of sexual commerce during pregnancy on the moral character of the child in utero, and may have frequent occasion to do so in time to come, it may be well to state more fully my meaning.

I suppose it to be an incontrovertible fact, that the more the foetal existence is undisturbed, and the more the whole physical, mental and moral energies of the mother are concentrated on the new being, the greater the probability that the latter will be reinstated, in due time, in the Divine image. The child whose energies are half robbed or destroyed ere he sees the light, will be likely to come forth upon the stage of life in such a debilitated or unbalanced state of body and mind as will render him a more ready slave to his own appetites and passions. Christianity may claim such individuals, no doubt, as they pass on in the journey of life; but its claims are not very greatly honored, nor the cause they would sustain greatly promoted, when their vitals have been sapped and drained and eaten out at the very threshold of their foetal existence.

It has sometimes been objected to the views which have been made prominent in this chapter, that parturition is much more easy and natural in those instances where the sexual instinct has not been wholly neglected during the period of pregnancy. But this opinion is one that will not stand the test of truth.

Some fifteen or twenty years ago, when I began to

press the claims of this subject upon the public mind, I received a long letter from a scientific gentleman, then in Europe, opposing, in some of its particulars, the doctrine of non-intercourse which I had been promulgating, and presenting what he believed to be a substantial reason for his opposition, namely, that it rendered parturition less difficult.

To me, it appeared quite sufficient to meet his objection with the following considerations:—

It has occasionally happened, in almost every age and country, that young, unmarried women have become mothers, and borne children, when the only sexual embrace they ever received was at the time of the conception of their illegitimate offspring.

Now if the above objection of my friend and correspondent were good and valid, we should naturally expect that these victims of weakness and seduction would have had more difficult or, at least, more prolonged labor than other women of the same age and circumstances. But the contrary is found to be much nearer the truth. The labor of these individuals is generally easy; at least, comparatively. In some instances their sufferings have been so trifling and their confinement so short, that their nearest neighbors have been utterly ignorant of their condition. Or if their illness for a day or two has been observed, it has been attributed, by others, to a cold or a "sick head-ache." They have even, like the wives of some of the American savages, on occasions, been delivered almost alone, and have covered, or attempted to cover, their shame, by destroying their offspring before enough of the world knew they had been mothers, to be able to testify against them.

For the general truth of the foregoing statement I have it in my power, most unfortunately, to appeal to nearly every densely populated neighborhood, even of our own comparatively virtuous and happy United America. In these neighborhoods may be found, in nearly every instance, some two or three, or perhaps half a dozen, aged individuals, who, from personal observation or well-authenticated report, will testify to the truth of my assertions.

The very common belief suggested by my correspondent is a weak one; and I should have passed it by unnoticed had it not been adopted by many sensible, and not a few intelligent, people who ought to know better; by those persons even, occasionally, who have made large claims to the knowledge of physiology and hygiene.

It has even been claimed by men in a position as responsible as that of a college professorship, that we go "too fast and too far" when we assume that the benevolent Creator of the sexes, in their original formation, ever contemplated such a prolonged season of non-intercourse of the sexes as is indicated by the general tenor of the reasonings of this chapter. Such prolonged abstinence, we are told, tends to alienate the feelings, if not to open the way to suspicions of infidelity. Frequent indulgence of this appetite, in married life, said one of these individuals, at least so frequent as to prevent certain evils to which an apostle refers, in writing to the Corinthians, is *endearing*. No doubt. But what is the kind of endearment? Does it have affinity to the spiritual nature, or is it merely instinctive? There is abroad, in vulgar life, a similar saying with regard to the lowest, most grovelling, and most filthy of domestic animals — that sleeping together makes them love each other!

The wife of a minister of the gospel, in one of our large cities committed suicide, a few years ago, in her own sleeping chamber. Some of the fancied wise ones of her neighborhood, in their very superficial search for the cause of so strange an event, believed they discovered it in a supposed alienation of feeling, induced by a pledge of herself and her husband to total abstinence for a few weeks, for the very simple and praiseworthy object of being able to do more for others. They were engaged heart and hand in a benevolent enterprise of very great magnitude and importance. Her death, it seems, took place in about six weeks after their separation.

Now it is one of the most common occurrences in the world — in these days of busy enterprise — for husbands and wives to separate for business or amusement, not merely six weeks, but as many months. Are these cases attended with an undue proportion of suicides? It would be difficult to prove this. It is even highly probable that there are fewer, than in other circumstances.

Let a maritime county in Massachusetts — that of

Barnstable — be called to the stand, on this occasion. The writer happens to be acquainted with a single neighborhood of that county, in which there are no less than thirty-five ship masters — men with families — besides a large number of common seamen, in similar circumstances. But it would be difficult to hear of a single suicide in all that region.

Only one more objection will be noticed at present. An aged and excellent deacon of a church in Connecticut, in a very valuable letter written many years since, took the position that God did not intend for the brutes as much of mere animal enjoyment as for man, the *nobler* animal. This is conjectural. It may or may not be so. It is certainly *possible* that more of sensual enjoyment is allotted to man in his disciplinary state, as an earnest of that higher, and nobler, and more scriptural enjoyment, which is in reserve for him when this corruptible shall have put on incorruption, and this mortal shall have put on immortality. It is, at least a pleasant *speculation*.

And yet I doubt, after all, whether these speculations — agreeable as they may be to many — are of much consequence. Had they not been the sober and dispassionate convictions of a most excellent follower of Christ, I should have been inclined to refer them to a very different source from that whence I now know them to have emanated. They would grace, far better, a shrewd apology for excessive amativeness.

Besides, whatever weight such speculations may

have had on the minds of others — and whatever of weight they really possess — is generally set to the credit of sexual indulgence generally; and not merely during the period of pregnancy. The subject was introduced in this place, as a mere matter of convenience.

The doctrine which I am defending in this chapter will meet with the strongest opposition from feeling — not from argument. It is so, generally, with anything which goes against the *propensities*. Convince men against their stomachs, and it is no conviction at all, practically. The stomach will over-ride all decisions of the higher court of judicature, the head. Paul himself, in his day, spoke of those individuals — and they are as numerous in these days as they ever were — whose God was no higher than the upper portion of the human abdomen. See Phil. iii., 19.

Is it so, then, can it be so, some reader will be likely to say, that a total and unqualified non-intercourse is the great law of human pregnancy — and that, too, without a solitary exception? Is that your exact meaning?

It is not precisely what I have affirmed; though it comes tolerably near the truth. According to the testimony of analogy and facts — and according to the general tenor and spirit of Christianity and science this must be the general rule. But almost all general rules have their exceptions; and there may be one or two in the present case. Let us briefly attend to them.

Woman, as is well known, in a natural state—unperverted, unseduced, and healthy — seldom, if ever, makes any of those advances, which clearly indicate sexual desire; and for this very plain reason that she does not feel them. I have even known of two or three most excellent female heads of large families, who *never* felt them. Such at least is their testimony.

On the contrary, not only before marriage, but during its first weeks and months, and through life, woman is to be *won*. And yet there are a few exceptions amounting in all probability to *diseased* cases. One of these, most certainly, is of this description. In it, the natural course of things is entirely reversed. — The following are the two most striking cases of diseased female amativeness with which I am acquainted.

In nervous women, at certain times, and under circumstances of pregnancy, it occasionally happens that the female appetite becomes erratic, and makes unusual, and in themselves considered, very objectionable demands. Distant articles of food or drink, or strange medicated mixtures, become the object of desire to an extent whose intenseness has long been characterized, or indicated, by the word *longing*.

This longing has been variously regarded and treated, both by the husband and the wife herself. In some instances the erratic demand has been most rigidly, not to say superstitiously complied with, even at the risk of affecting, injuriously, the health, both of the mother and her offspring. It has even been supposed, by a few, that both the mother and her offspring would be seriously injured — especially the latter — without them. In other instances, the desire is laughed at, both by the husband and the other friends; and unless the wife is made of adamant, or is able to join in a laugh against herself, she often becomes a serious sufferer.

Now these erratic appetites are not to be despised or trifled with, on the one hand; nor wholly and unreservedly yielded to, on the other. Woman should fully understand their cause, and endeavor to act the part of reason as much as possible. What can be done, without too much inconvenience, and without too much of opposition to the laws of health and life, should be done; what it seems necessary to dispense with, should, in the true spirit of Christianity, be given up.

The husband and friends should have the same feelings, and should pursue a similar course. Nature should not be trampled on, I say, on the one hand; nor over-indulged or pampered, on the other. It should be understood that disease, or at least debility, is at the foundation of all these things. It is usually quite enough for the hardiest and healthiest female constitution to go through with the trials of gestation and child bearing, without faltering; and when the system falters, as a whole, it is not strange that the appetites should sympathize in the general embarrassment. In this condition of things, the appetite which God, in his wise Providence, has established within us, as a means of perpetuating the species, becomes erratic, at least occasionally, as well as the rest.

Woman, though before reserved, modest, and even distant, becomes now, on occasions, open, bold, and forward. — I say *on occasions*, because it is exceedingly seldom, even in those individuals who are constitutionally most inclined to it.

Under these circumstances, it may and does become a grave question which will be productive of most harm, to repel the diseased appetite or to yield, temporarily — perhaps in a single instance — to its demands. So far as the question relates to the mere health of the female, in itself considered, I have not a doubt that such an occasional indulgence would be favorable. It is quite another question whether the child will suffer less or more from a persevering self-denial, amid feelings of continued uneasiness and unhappiness; or whether, as a choice of evils, the contrary course, in an instance or two, should be pursued.

The common idea that the child in utero suffers, if the mother's desires are not gratified, is correct, in a certain sense; and yet, in other points of view, incorrect. It is certainly true that if the mother suffers, whether that suffering arises from one cause or another, the child is not so well sustained, as the consequence, in the uterus. But when this doctrine is carried to the extent of some; when we are told that if the mother longs for a particular fruit, the product of a distant land, which cannot be obtained, or is refused something which might be procured for her, the child will be marked with that particular article, or will come into the world with a half insane and quite insatiable craving for it, we are, as friends of sound science, compelled to demur.

There is a second exception to the general rule of non-intercourse during pregnancy. This is more obviously a case of disease than the former; for the disease and the actual condition of the diseased parts are now well understood. It is what is called, in books, nymphomania.

It may be said — I suppose it will be said — that women who are affected with this troublesome complaint, ought not to enter the bonds of matrimony. This may be true; nevertheless they sometimes do. Indeed it is a very commonly received opinion that matrimony is a cure for several diseases; and for this among the rest. And would it not be very unreasonable to expect women who have never been informed on this subject, to rise much above the level of vulgar prejudices? The husband, moreover, in these days, who finds himself united, for life, to a woman whose only defect or weakness is a slight nymphomania, may think himself quite fortunate.

It is a curious fact, by the way, that mothers are sometimes much more anxious to see their sickly, or at least feeble daughters settled in life, than their more healthy ones. The reasons for this are various — but I cannot present them, in detail. It is sufficient for our purpose that I have stated, in broad and unmistakable terms, the existing fact, and alluded faintly to what may be one of the principal.

Now if, beyond these two exceptions to the general law of non-intercourse, there are any others, I must frankly confess that I know not what they are. But it is not my object, in the preparation of this work, to say everything which can be said on the physiology and hygiene of marriage; but rather to present what I have been taught, by a long course of reading, observation, and experience, to be true.

I am fully aware that it is not easy for human nature, as it now is, to receive some of the doctrines I have here inculcated, especially those of the present chapter. Our sex, in general, have been so trained as to entertain a very different view of woman from that which I have been led to embrace. Women have rights of various kinds; among these are some few which their most renowned champions have not yet ventured — at least in public halls, and on public platforms — to claim for them. They have the right of asserting and maintaining, against all aggression, their own *health* and the health of those whom God has, in more than one sense, committed to their charge.

But my business with the young is only half accomplished when I have merely asserted and unfolded the laws of pregnancy, and told them *what should not be done*. There are sins of omission, in this world, as well as of commission. There are things to be done by us, the professed lords of the creation,* during a

* I do not mean, by this, a reproach on our own sex, so much as a hint with regard to the kind of rule or dominion which is delegated to men by Divine appointment, not only

season when those who are constitutionally weaker than ourselves, bear for our race, by Divine appointment, a burden which we cannot bear for them, if we would do it. There is much to be done, if we would not only encourage but assist in the great work of training up a generation that will coöperate with the Son of God, in the redemption — body, soul and spirit — of a fallen race.

We should be at least as earnest in seeking woman's comfort and happiness, during pregnancy, as we have before been in seeking our own. In saying this, however, I do not associate with the word *happiness* any of those mawkish ideas which many husbands do. It is one thing to attempt to make woman happy by treating her as a mere doll, only to make her still more a plaything than before; and quite another thing to treat her as a woman, a wife, and a Christian.

It is really too trifling for a man five or six feet high to amuse himself, or think to perform the duties he owes to his wife under the most trying circumstances in which female nature can be placed, merely by presenting her, from time to time, with those petty trifles, and those alone, which, after all, only minister to the clamorous demands of already perverted appetites and fallen tastes, and render those tastes and appetites still

in his creation, but in the ordinary ways of Providence. Man is to rule, as a good king should rule, by conferring favor on his subjects, as being weaker than he, and by advancing their interests to the full extent of his power, in all sorts of known ways for promoting their happiness.

more perverted and clamorous. This is an extreme almost as silly as that of despising and attempting to turn out of doors those erratic appetites which I have, in the foregoing pages, described.

He who would make his wife, both *as* a wife, and in prospect as a mother, truly and really happy, should labor, in the first place, to make her as healthy as possible, both in body and mind. This, during the season of pregnancy, is not, always, an easy thing. In the great work of establishing a new being, at the expense, so to call it, of a delicate and perhaps enfeebled female frame, nature too often cowers; and it is hardly to be wondered at, if in these circumstances, she should feel, in an unusual degree, the need of aid and sympathy.

Woman, in these circumstances, above all other things except kind aid and sympathy, needs pure air by night and by day; and abundant, but not too violent physical and mental exercise. She also needs a full supply — but by no means an over supply, — of good nutritious food. But nutritious food and stimulating food are by no means identical, though not a few seem to suppose they are. The latter would be as injurious as the former is beneficial.

I have alluded to mental exercise. The tendencies in woman, during pregnancy, are so many of them downward, towards the land of melancholy if not of despondency, that it may sometimes require a little effort to give the mental powers just the right employment, and prevent the mind from pursuing a mill-horse track, and preying upon itself. Many seem to think that it they walk just so far every day, say to such a tree, or house, or hill, they have done all they can do. And yet it is quite possible they have come far short of the full benefit which exercise is calculated to impart, when the mind too, has change, as well as the body.

On this account it might be well for all, especially for all women in pregnancy, in going abroad for exercise, to have associates with whom they may hold agreeable and cheerful conversation. But at any rate, and at all hazards, there should be great cheerfulness and happy is the husband who is disposed to aid in keeping a wife cheerful, even if it costs some sacrifice.

It is by no means intended that a husband should give himself up to the work of endeavoring to render his wife cheerful during her "appointed time," and do nothing else. With at least one warlike nation of which we read, it was deemed proper for the young husband to remain with and comfort his wife, after marriage, a whole year, before he was liable to be drawn into the military service of his country; but such usages, nationally or individually, are not common. Such facts, whenever and wherever we can glean them up, are suggestive, but they are hardly entitled to higher consideration.

We must draw towards a close of this long chapter, not because our subject is exhausted, or because the objections which might be urged against the views herein presented have all been answered; but because it was determined, from the first, not to be led aside into collateral subjects, or even into very much of detail on the main topics. There is room, however, for one or two thoughts more.

One of these is the following. Is it not surprising that nature, unperverted, the female nature I mean, should not have taught us, long before now, one important part of our duty as regards physical marriage? The very fact that no advances are ordinarily made by females during pregnancy, even where the temperament of the individual, to say nothing of diseased tastes and tendencies, would incline her in that direction, should, with all sensible men, have much weight.

The other thought has relation to the purity of the air in our sleeping rooms. If any adult person in the wide world needs pure air, it is pregnant woman. She needs it for her own sake; she needs it still more for her offspring. I have said that she must, at all hazards, be cheerful; but who can be cheerful without good air in their lungs, and in sufficient quantity?

Two reasons exist which render it necessary that particular attention should be paid to the matter of pure air, during pregnancy. One of these grows out of the fact that female dress tends to cramp and embarrass the lungs to an extent which, in any circumstances, very much interferes with the needful work of renewing the blood in the lungs. Some pregnant women, when they are panting for breath, loosen their dress, at least occasionally; but if they are to be seen out of their own family circle, conventional law, in other words, fashion, usually prevails, and the screws are re-applied. The fact that women dress too tightly, now-a-days, may be questioned by some, but is, unhappily, pretty well attested. Then, again, in the most favorable moments of advanced pregnancy, the chest is not so well expanded as usual by reason of the upward pressure of the abdominal contents. Here is a general and strong reason for extra effort, by night and by day, in order that the diminished quantity of air which is inhaled, in a case where an increased amount is imperatively needed, may be as pure as possible.

Now is this point secured when woman is secluded too much, and especially when she is confined to hot rooms and impure air? Is our duty to her duly performed, — aye, and our duty to our offspring too, — when we do nothing to drag her forth beyond the inner walls of the domestic sanctuary?

Are we doing our duty when we suffer her to sleep in a narrow, unventilated bed-room, especially during the later months of her seclusion? And does it add to the purity of the air she is to breathe to have others occupying the same bed, and using up one half or more of the natural supply of oxygen which God, in his Providence, had designed for her?

It does not follow, as a matter of absolute necessity, that a husband shall sleep at a distance. Woman needs sympathy, above all, during pregnancy. He may have his bed in the same room, if the room is large; or, if not, a door or two may perhaps be thrown open to form a channel of intercommunication, as well as to secure a measure of ventilation.

I might say a good deal of other evils to which a sleeping-partner exposes the female; and still more her offspring. There are many ways of accidentally inflicting violence, in these circumstances, which might result in still-birth or abortion, if nothing worse. But perhaps I have said enough. Should not a word to the wise, on such a subject, be sufficient?

CHAPTER X.

CRIMES WITHOUT NAME.

For nearly everything valuable in civic life, we are compelled to submit to a greater or less degree of taxation; though this apparent drawback upon our enjoyment is usually least perceptible in the case of real necessaries, such as air, water, clothing, and plain food. Yet even air and water, and plain food, can hardly be obtained without some pains-taking.

This almost universal taxation, though in many cases slight in amount, and perhaps so far removed from tyranny as to be usually fraught with blessings in disguise, is heavier just in proportion as we rise higher in the region of present indulgence. The taxes of luxurious eating and drinking are greater than those which are levied on plainer viands. Nevertheless, mankind usually prefer the former to the latter, even with the taxes. Or, what is nearer strict truth, instead of honestly complying with the stern demands, and fulfilling the exact conditions of a known law, they seize and appropriate to their own use the more doubtful pleasure, and then evade, if they can, the payment of the tax.

Every man knows, or ought to know, that the great object of the sexual function is the reproduction of the species; and though not all the seed which is cast into the human soil is expected to germinate and grow, yet when it does spring up and bring forth, he is bound to take care of it; and the younger and more delicate the germ, or the shoot, the greater is his obligation to rear it and nurture it, even till it reaches maturity.

This, I have by figure, called a tax. Is such taxation tyrannous? It is not deemed burdensome and tyrannous to be compelled to take care of the young shoot in the vegetable world; nor the young calf or lamb in the animal world. At least, it should not be so. These we watch over, and with pleasure, from germination to maturity. Or if it were possible for us to feel such cares to be burdensome at the time, the usefulness of the crop, when matured, would be apt to make us forget the tax we had paid. Is the promise of the future, in the case of human reproduction, of less value?

Some appear to regard it so; indeed, many do.— They wish for full liberty to scatter their seed; it is a pleasure to them, a luxury to which they seem to think themselves entitled; but they do not wish to have a crop. It would be burdensome to them. A mow of wheat or rye, or a bin of corn they would highly prize; but a family of children they do not want. The burden of rearing young immortals would be a taxation so tyrannous that they could not endure it.

Hence it is that ways, almost innumerable, are devised for evading nature's laws altogether. Some of these ways are more, others less objectionable; but they all partake in greater or less degree of the same character. They are all evasions. They are all criminal, even though they should be, as they seem to be, crimes without names.

Some twenty or twenty-five years ago, a physician of New England, of much greater practical skill than strict integrity, especially towards God, became the author of a small pocket volume, with a very inviting title, whose avowed object was to teach people, both in married life and elsewhere, the art of gratifying the sexual appetite without the necessity of progeny. His book had a wide circulation. I have found it in nearly every part of our wide-spread country.

It was the more successful, no doubt, from the fact that the author declared his chemical mixture or lotion to be not only certain in its preventive effects, if applied immediately, but entirely uninjurious to the delicate tissues against which it was injected. It is in vogue, even now, in many parts of our country, and is highly prized. They, who have tried it, usually regard it as entirely certain in its effects; though I have reason to doubt the soundness of this conclusion.

I am well acquainted with one whole maritime county of New England, whose husbands and wives, to a very large extent, do not wish to have issue. The husbands are, for the most part, and for the far greater part of the year, absent. They are not willing to subject the party at home to confinement, in solitude; nor even to the trouble of rearing children without the co-operation and aid of a companion. Nor is the wife who remains at home much more willing to be subjected to these evils. There may be present, there doubtless are, some of the other motives which so extensively prevail; such as the love of pleasure, a regard to economy, or the fear of absolute poverty; but the ostensible motives are a regard to each others' feelings and convenience.

Now among the means used to prevent the fulfilment of the great command, " Increase and multiply and replenish the earth," by the comparatively simple people I have just mentioned, is Dr. ——'s chemical lotion. And, as I said before, it usually succeeds; but then, I have also heard of occasional failures.

Frequent indulgence, as a preventive of conception, has been already incidentally mentioned. But it is not only true that prostitutes seldom conceive; those who pursue a course of prostitution within the pale of matrimony come under the same general law. Now this matrimonial prostitution, one half the year, namely, the winter, is considerably frequent, everywhere; but particularly in the region I have just mentioned.

How far this indulgence is *intended* as a preventive of conception, I am not quite certain. It is so frequently followed by the chemical preparation I have described, as well as by a degree of violence and carelessness which, if not intentional, is greatly unfavorable, that it is not easy to know how far particular results are the consequence of concerted action. But however this may be, it is most certain that foetal germination, growth, and development require quiet; and so does the well-being of the mother herself.

Another course of conduct which, sometimes from ignorance, sometimes from intention, has either a preventive or an abortive effect, is going abroad a good deal to parties of pleasure, especially by night. So far as mere cheerfulness is concerned, the going abroad is of happy tendency; but the excitement which usually, or at least frequently accompanies balls, assemblies, concerts, and all pleasure parties, especially where large numbers congregate; is always injurious. And then, above all, the physical excitements, the bad air, high-seasoned food, exciting drink, and late hours, saying nothing now of other irregularities, are, if possible, much more hazardous than the mental ones. If there should be no considerable violence or concussion, there is a tendency, as a whole, to injure the mother, and, still more, the offspring; and not a few know this, and govern themselves accordingly. I have, as a physician, known families in which it was believed the mother made special efforts by jumping, on these occasions, especially at the point of extreme fatigue, in hope of destroying what previous efforts had failed to prevent.

It not unfrequently happens that several of the causes I have been enumerating are united. In such cases, conception is more certainly prevented, or early abortion more certainly secured, than where only one cause of destruction is operative. Thus, late evening parties, as I have before intimated, and carelessless, with frequent sexual indulgence, are very generally brought to bear, in solid phalanx, against the struggling tendency to life and light with almost as much certainty of success as that two and two make four.

Some few there are who prevent conception by violent labor. They do it, I mean, intentionally. The least fear of what may happen almost makes them rave, as with habitual anger. Indeed, so far as I have observed, most women are unwilling to *bear* children. Most, it is true, are anxious to be mothers; but only a small number are willing to pay the price. How few act, in this matter, with any sense of duty, or any proper regard to principle?

How many, especially in the lower walks of life, shall we find laboring with unusual energy, when a recent suspicion has arisen in their minds; and persisting in their labor, even to exertions which are violent! And this general disposition to avoid conception and pregnancy seems to me greatly increasing.

Now if to some or all the causes, above-mentioned, which have an agitating tendency on the human system, we add prolonged violent efforts, hard lifting, or straining, who does not know that the results aimed at are pretty sure to follow, and are, in some women, quite inevitable?

Thousands, that might otherwise have lived, have been destroyed by violent motion and concussions of various sorts. In certain portions of our country tradition has at hand a long list of certain measures for securing a result which is, by many, deemed so important.

But of all the measures for accomplishing these results which I have called *crimes without name*, none are more common, I think, than the use of poison of one kind or another, and that of instruments; and certainly none are more reprehensible. True it is, that if done with the same intention, crime is crime, at any period of fœtal development; and not less so at conception. Still there is something peculiarly shocking in those cases of destruction which approximate to maturity of the embryo, especially when the results are accomplished by poison, or by surgical instruments.

The public, as a general thing, are not aware — perhaps it may be well that they are not so — to what an extent this violence against Nature and Nature's God, is carried on in our country; nor how respectable are the names of some of the agents in these diabolical results.

True it is that many who find themselves pregnant resort to tradition and household practice for what they call relief. Some field, or swamp, or grove contains the needful poison; and forthwith it is swallowed Sometimes life is destroyed as the result; — I mean, now, the life of the principal offender — but it happens, much more frequently, that she escapes with less injury than her offspring.

But there are physicians, male and female — physicians they style themselves, though sometimes such by the appointment of a college for the education of horses or horse doctors, if any — in many parts of the country, whose counsels may be had for a very small sum; or, if not, *for a large one!* To these men, when household prescriptions fail, it is not unusual for application to be made.

In the progress of operation by these physicians, real or pretended — whether male or female, and in city or country — it sometimes happens that owing to want of skill, or to the intrinsic difficulties of the case, immediate death occurs. In these circumstances it is only necessary to use a little of what quacks call management. The underground railroad from the "doctor's" house to the late home of the deceased, is no longer or more difficult than the underground road which brought her to the bench of the operator. And every reader knows how easy it is in these days to announce "sudden death;" and the public swallow it all down at once. Mankind on particular occasions, and in certain matters where there is a sort of common concern and common guilt, are wonderfully gullible.

I wish it were practicable to obtain the statistics of these *crimes without names*, and publish them to the world. They must come to light here or hereafter Is it not just as well that they should come out here?

Let us call to our aid for once, a little imagination. A table embracing the elements to which I refer may be supposed something like the following:

Destroyed, yearly, by means of a certain book,

clandestinely circulated .... ten thousands.
Destroyed by too frequent intercourse .. thousands.
Destroyed by careless intercourse ...... thousands.
Destroyed by violent intentional efforts .. thousands.
Destroyed by accidental means......... hundreds.
Destroyed by poisoning — foreign and domestic .... ten thousands.
Destroyed by instrumental violence .... hundreds.
Destroyed by over working .... hundreds

I am not a little ashamed to own that among the men — and I fear women too — who aid in this nefarious work, a work for which Herod himself might have blushed for guilt and shame, are a few who have received the diplomas of other colleges besides *horse* colleges. What will not men do — beings in the shape of men, I mean — for money? Such individuals ought to be expelled from every respectable body of men with whom they may chance to be connected, if not from the world, itself. In truth, I know of very few crimes for which capital punishment should be inflicted, if not for this.

But if our physicians, men who have reduced themselves to a depth of infamy of which Milton's rebel angels who fell "nine days," might be ashamed — if these deserve hanging, what shall be done with our Madam Restells and a host of other madams in our large cities and elsewhere, who make good the poet's stigma: —

"A shameless woman is the worst of men!"

But I turn from the detail of these "crimes without name" in disgust, and almost in indignation, and pass to consider some of the effects of this violence on the mother and her offspring generally. For it is not the dead alone that we mourn, in this connection; the living, too, are sufferers. I will illustrate, and endeavor to prove.

It is sometimes said — and by many it appears to be believed — that the mothers and wives in the particular maritime district to which I have but just now referred, are as old, now a days, at forty-five, as they were half a century ago at sixty years of age. This premature age is, I know, ascribed by many, to their anxiety — and sometimes excessive grief — about their distant sons, and brothers, and husbands. But how can it be known, by those who entertain such notions, that the cause to which I have directed your attention, has had nothing to do with it?

But proof is not wanting in the case. Among the inhabitants aforesaid is an aged pair, who are not only themselves prematurely old, but whose children, too, are diseased and feeble. This now aged couple set out, in life, with a general determination to have no family. The measures adopted to prevent such a result were those which they deemed most justifiable, and most safe. And yet despite of all their efforts, they have had — I believe now have — no less than six living children. And yet, as I said before, they have none of them, much hardihood. The stoutest and strongest has been obliged to pass his winters in a southern climate.

And now, reader, perhaps with your want of experience in human nature and things, I shall somewhat surprise you when I tell you that I was once consulted, as a medical man, by the parties most concerned in this remarkable case, in order to know whether I believed it possible that the feebleness of six children could be owing to the preventive efforts, of various kinds, which had been made by the parents.

Here was what I regard as the concession of plain unsophisticated common sense to a well known physiological fact. Of course you need not *guess* at my reply to the inquiry. No child could be as healthy, other things and circumstances being equal, who was born in spite of parental efforts to prevent it, as the child of parents who had made no such attempts to thwart the tendencies of Nature to reproduction. And I ought not to close my remarks under this head without saying that I found occasional instances of this sort, all over the aforesaid maritime district, and some even elsewhere.

Another thing, too, must not be omitted. In no other region that I have visited, not wholly given up to the crowded merchant and manufacturer, have I found so large a proportion of the population either consumptive or scrofulous, as in the one we are now considering. But of the connection direct and indirect, between consumption, and sexual error and abuse, I have said something already.

If you wish to see a truly healthy family of children accompanied by a mother who is apparently little older or less vigorous than they, just go with me to a certain house, within the circle of my acquaintance, where there are twelve or fourteen children of various ages from two upward — just about two years apart, and all born at the appointed time, and without any manual interference.

Some may be inclined to inquire whether there are no parental conditions and circumstances which would both justify and require a departure from Nature's general plan. Must she who has it not in her power to nurse her own children, though in tolerable bodily health, be in every particular obedient to the great command, "Increase and multiply?" Must she who is insane or consumptive? Must they who have been reduced as a family, — perhaps by no fault of their own — to sudden poverty, the most abject?

These inquiries are appropriate and important. My reply shall be as brief as the nature of the case will admit.

With regard to the first mentioned case it may be remarked that there is found, here and there, a mother who without the ability to nurse her own offspring, has yet become the female head of a large and comparatively healthy family. Such a result, as we plainly see, is far enough from being impossible; and yet it is not to be relied on, as a general rule. Without doubt the general law is that a mother shall nurse her own children, or not bear them.

As to the other two inquiries, the answer is more difficult; and I must candidly confess myself unable.

at present, to say what is the exact rule of duty. If two young persons come together in married life, fully aware of their tendencies to disease — and I see not why a courtship conducted on sound principles, and under the general direction of wise parents, should not give the parties, respectively, this knowledge — and the laws of physiology and hygiene clearly point to a strong probability that severe or dangerous disease will be transmitted to offspring, should they have any, I can scarcely entertain a doubt that it is their duty to remain childless. It would be a preferable course, however, for such parties not to marry. We have no right, with our eyes open, to propagate a race with every reasonable prospect of its being a sickly one.

There are one or two measures which might be adopted for the prevention of offspring, which, though perhaps open to criticism, in some few particulars, are, nevertheless, to be regarded, on the whole, in a somewhat different light.

A measure of the animal or sexual enjoyment pertaining to the sexual embrace, may be obtained by a species of self-denial on the part of the husband, which though it should be, in its essential form, like that of Onan, would be without his particular form of guilt. Masturbation and Onanism, as the careful reader will see, are not by any means the same thing; though such was, formerly, the prevailing impression.

Suppose, however, it should be doubted by any individual, whether he possesses the power of self-control to the full extent of the patriarch I have mentioned, and suppose, too, its propriety should be doubted, it is nevertheless obvious that one thing more remains. It is a measure recommended by many judicious writers, and certainly entitled to a moment's consideration.

It seems to be a well known physiological law that conception cannot take place at every period of female life between the catamenial discharges; but only during the first fortnight, or as some say, the first eight days which immediately follow the cessation of the menses. If, therefore, we deny ourselves, during a full fortnight as above mentioned, no subsequent intercourse, up to the commencement of the next catamenial discharge, can possibly be productive.

You will observe that I have been stating in the last paragraph, a generally received opinion; and not a mere surmise of my own. Whether the course which is thus indicated is right or not, is quite another question. I will only say that if it is *not* right, many an individual in this world we occupy, who wishes to do right at all hazards and all sacrifices, is after all, in this particular, still wrong.

In any event one grand, final resort remains, still — that of refraining from the sexual embrace altogether. Some have taken this course. Others have feared to adopt a course so rigid, on others' account. A still greater number have refused to do it on their own account. They have not been quite satisfied. They have doubted its righteousness.

I will only add, at present, the language of Paul —

leaving to others to make their own application; —
"Let every man be fully persuaded in his own mind."
"He that doubteth is condemned if he eat."

CHAPTER XI.

THE LAWS OF LACTATION OR NURSING.

Dr. Loudon, an eminent British writer, maintains that children ought not to be entirely weaned from their mother till they are two years of age.

This decision, of very high authority, may perhaps answer for the social latitude and longitude of England; but it cannot do so well for the United States of America. Here, not a few mothers, who call themselves healthy, would suffer, more or less, and some very seriously, by extending the period of lactation much beyond one year. And the number is exceedingly small of those who can nurse a child as many as two whole years.

Suppose, however, there were no objections to such a long period of lactation, on the part of the mother — would it be well for the child? And then again, as we are told by our physiologists that the sexual embrace should be postponed during this period, is there no objection to be derived from this consideration? Man, it will be said, cannot forget always, that he is man — certainly not two or three years at a time;

must there not, then, be some mistake in the matter? And what is the exact law?

With regard to that part of the objection which affirms that the law is too rigid for man to receive, as he now is, I suppose, in reality, we have nothing to say. If it is law, the great Creator made it so, and not I, or any physiologist. We have but to ascertain that a thing is really law, and then yield our hearty assent to it, let it affect our present feelings and pleasures as it may.

But herein is the question to be settled — what *is* the law? My own views do not entirely accord with those that would seem to lie on the surface of the foregoing. The extent of the period of lactation does not determine the limits of the period of non-intercourse of the sexes. That limit is to be determined much more by a reference to the condition of the infant's teeth.

I do not mean by this that as soon as the first teeth of the infant appear, we have full latitude given us to the indulgence of our passions and appetites; but only that this appearance indicates the commencement of a season in which sexual indulgence is not absolutely prohibited.

Some have placed this beginning period at the return of the menstrual discharge; which, as you know, usually disappears during pregnancy, and early lactation; but this seems to me too uncertain a point. Most persons like to have something more certain and definite. Some women, moreover, menstruate during the whole period of lactation, if not of pregnancy; while, in others, this function does not resume its wonted course till the child is entirely weaned, — whether this embraces a period of one or two years, or even longer.

It will be observed, however, that when I speak of the first dentition, as being the proper period for a recurrence to venereal pleasures, it is only, after all, by way of compromise. For, as it cannot come earlier, and as the period of pregnancy, and this early period of lactation, when taken together, include at least fourteen or fifteen consecutive months of non-intercourse, it appears to me that a species of compromise is, in the circumstances, quite justifiable. I mean just this: Although it is true that we are guided best by the catamenia, at least when that discharge ceases, yet a partial return to the sexual embrace at a period somewhat earlier than this usually happens after pregnancy, may be preferable, on the whole, to a more rigid adherence to the strictest letter and closest interpretation of physiological law.

But I may, perhaps, be asked by those whose opportunities for information on this subject have been more limited than others, why it is that non-intercourse is demanded during any period of lactation, except perhaps the very first month. They can understand, they may say, why the enfeebled state of the mother may forbid this during the first few weeks, but not afterward. The child is no longer a part of the mother, and can receive no injury, they add; and now if there is no objection on the part of either the mother or the child, whence comes any objection at all?

The reply to all this is, that though the child is no longer a part of the mother, *nominally*, yet it is so *really*. That is, it is so, to all practical intents and purposes; and as such, needs all the support which the most vigorous condition of body and mind both, in the mother, can impart. Sexual commerce, so far as the mother partakes in the act, deprives the child in her arms, or rather at her breast, of its rightful nourishment; and unless there is a natural superabundance of that nourishment, the child is as certainly robbed as if an attack had been made upon it on the highway. There may, it is true, be this difference in the two cases. The highway robber usually takes away nothing but our property; while the parental robber takes away his child's health. Even if it were pleaded that the mother furnished an over-abundant supply, it is still to be remembered that perchance the quality of the secretion from the breast might be impaired by sexual intercourse.

Now what would we say of a father who should, by force of arms, deprive his child, — a helpless infant child, — of his rightful title to property, real or personal? "Who steals my purse, steals trash;" we have again and again heard. But to steal from a child would be a crime. But how much more strange, — nay, how much more reprehensible, — the act on the part of a parent, who, with open eye and full consciousness of what he was doing, deprives his child of that constitutional health and vigor to which God, in his providence, has given him a good and valid and unalienable title?

Not only is every father bound not to *rob* his children of their property or their health, but to see that their just rights are conceded to them by others. More than even this might be said. He is bound to do all in his power to add to his child's estate, — especially in the matter of constitutional vigor, — to the full extent of his ability. This is to be brought about in several ways.

First, by avoiding the very common error of sleeping in the same bed with the mother and the child. I have urged this point of sleeping separately already, and given several reasons why it is objectionable during pregnancy; but other considerations come in here. God has made provision in the child's constitution for such a deficiency of oxygen as may enable it to sleep in the mother's bosom; yet he has not provided for that deficiency of this precious commodity, and that redundancy of carbonic acid gas, which will be found in a bed of only ordinary dimensions, in which there are two or three grown persons.

Secondly. We thus diminish the temptation — rather we prevent it — to rob the child, in a more direct manner. The heat of the bed, as well as other existing circumstances, where many living bodies are crowded together, is as unfavorable to self-denial as it is to health.

Thirdly. We should keep always before us, in mind, that we are to be the progenitors of a race, either of transgressors, or of those who obey in love — as numerous, perhaps, as Eve has been the mother of, up to this hour. But I have presented this main idea in another connection; and need not here repeat.

One objection, — one which to many will seem final and unanswerable, — will no doubt be made to the whole tenor of my reasoning, both in this, and chapters VII, and IX. It will be said that I require a degree of abstinence which human nature cannot bear, as it now is; and since God is the author of human nature, it is but a reasonable presumption that he has not so arranged things as to require of his creatures what is almost an impossibility.

Why, according to your views, it will be said, there are merely a few short intervals, at least this side of the age of forty-five or fifty years, when we may approach woman at all. She is not approachable till matrimony, of course; in this, all agree. Then she is to bear children, once in about two years, from twenty-two to forty-five; and pregnancy and lactation being seasons of non-intercourse, we have only nine months of every two years, during which, according to your views, she is at all accessible. But nine months for every two years under forty-five, give us an aggregate of only about ninety months. Can it be that this is an arrangement of Infinite Wisdom?

I might reply by saying that even at this rate, — and leaving unmentioned the period beyond forty-five or fifty, — much greater license is given us, than is given to the beasts that perish. Are we more brutal, — rather more truly animal, — than they? If not, why do we demand a more free use of what might be called the animal prerogative?

But however this may be, — for I do not lay claim to papal infallibility, — I greatly desire young men to be self-denying. Never did I stand by the bed-side of a dying man — and I have stood by the dying beds of many, — who lamented that he had not indulged, in a higher degree his animal nature. Often have I heard lamentations of entirely another character — regrets that the higher nature had not oftener gained a victory over the lower.

CHAPTER XII.

CRIMES THAT DESERVE NO NAME.

AMONG the numerous letters I have received on the same subject, — that which forms the leading topic of this chapter, — I select the following for insertion in this place, and for comment. It was received in the beginning of the year 1852, from a young woman in the very heart of New England. The apologies for addressing me on a subject of so delicate a nature, with preliminaries, I shall omit entirely; and proceed at once to the extracts.

"I think my difficulty is one of the uterus, combined with other weaknesses of similar location. I am now twenty-six years of age; have been a widow some years; have been troubled with a weakness since the first year of my marriage."

In another letter, one which contains not a few repetitions, — a thing not at all unusual in such cases, — she writes thus : —

"I am twenty-six years of age. I was married and left a widow while young and very ignorant, under circumstances the most painful."

Now every medical man who receives such letters

as these, knows, too well, what they mean; though to others the "circumstances" described as being "most painful," and the "weakness" which had troubled her 'from the first year of her marriage," might mean one thing or another, according to the measure of general intelligence on such subjects. So might the following farther extracts from her letters, which serve to show how deep was the anguish of soul which she endured in her attempts to reveal to a stranger her difficulties. She was suffering as the consequence of a "crime which deserves no name."

"I am an ardent, impulsive creature, possessing a nervous, sanguine temperament, naturally cheerful and equable; but rendered, by sickness, irritable and capricious. I came of a long-lived family; and for that reason I fear I shall die of some lingering disease. My mind is made up in regard to the future, so that my hopes of heaven are pleasant. The most I dread is the struggle in separating from life. I fear consumption so much that were I convinced it was fastened upon me, and were I not restrained by a strong moral influence, I might be tempted to commit a crime which could not be forgiven."

Another extract reveals more deeply still, if possible, the intensity of her mental sufferings.

"I am unaccountable to myself. I think, sir, that my mental disturbances greatly impair my health. Imagine, sir, a well-built ship, having powerful machinery, but without a pilot on board to direct it to its destined port! I see, by your letter, you understand me."

One more extract, still: —

"I feel a universal languor. I am, at times, unconscious. I feel dead to all things. There seems a loss of vitality. At other times, I feel a sense of suffocation. All these feelings are extreme; because I am one of those who possess very strong feelings, both by inheritance and temperament.

"I met the other day with a slight from a friend, a lady, which caused such excessive grief that I have ever since been suffering from influenza."

And now, young men who read this, what think you was the cause of all this suffering, both real and imaginary — for imaginary evils are sometimes quite as hard to bear, as real ones? My visits, subsequently, to this poor woman, left no room for doubt. She revealed to me, as to a father, no less than a physician, facts which I had already expected — such facts, I am sorry to say, as are not, by any means, unfrequent — whose detail, as I suppose, had an influence on my mind in leading me to write this very chapter. By her marriage to a young man whom she loved, she had contracted a disease, which however justly inflicted on him, should never have been communicated to her. Heaven's decrees and laws may sometimes seem rigid; but Heaven itself never appears to have made provision for such punishment as this. It punishes woman as well as man, for sinning out of wedlock; but virtue and vice are alike assailed within the pale of the marriage institution, when such wretches as the husband of this young woman come to be invested with power.

Were this young woman a solitary sufferer from this source, I would not have said a single word. Were she even but one among a dozen or a score, I might have hesitated. But, alas! thousands suffer in like manner. In one of our most sober and even most refined cities of comparatively virtuous New England, I have full and reliable evidence of the existence of this crime that deserves no name; and that, too, in many instances. But if the polite and highly cultivated city of twenty thousand inhabitants, is in this respect guilty, what are we to expect of such places as New York, Baltimore, New Orleans, Philadelphia, and fifty other considerable cities and towns, which I could name?

Nay, more than even this. While apologizing to my audience at the close of a lecture which had elicited a few passing remarks on this subject, and expressing the charitable hope that the remarks in such a quiet, industrious, and virtuous community were uncalled for, I have had the repeated assurance that *even there* crimes so undeserving of a name had found their way at least occasionally. We are sometimes compelled, in spite of ourselves and our charities, to subscribe to the declaration of eighteen hundred years ago, that "the whole world lieth in wickedness."

Here, for example, in central Massachusetts, was a young man of apparently good standing in society. I affirm this with substantial reasons; for otherwise I am sure he would not have ventured to address a young woman, who, to say the least, was respectable and intelligent. But he addressed her — probably loved her, and offered her his hand. The feeling was reciprocated — the union, in due time, was consummated. But he was suffering under the effects of venereal disease. Of his guilt in its contraction, 1 will not say a word. He had the disease; this is enough, and too much. He gave it to an inoffensive woman — one, moreover, whom he professed to love, and, as I said before, probably *did* love. Do crimes like these deserve a name? And do those who commit them with open eyes — and with open eyes they must do it, if done at all — deserve a place in decent society? And if capital punishment, by hanging, shooting, etc., is to be banished from among us, should we not at least have some lazar house — some leprous community — some Botany Bay — whither to send such criminals as might, perchance, disgrace a common halter, or even a guillotine?

But I must not lose patience, I suppose, in the review of crimes so horrid. If God does not strike dead the criminal, but suffers him to go on in his awful course of guilt, unscathed even by the forked lightning or the raging floods of burning lava, it becomes me — though I proclaim loud his guilt as a warning to others — to bow in silence, and await the punishment to be inflicted by Him who sits enthroned beyond the electric cloud, or the flaming and quivering volcano.

You will say; But perhaps the young man above mentioned, thought he was cured. The notion is certainly abroad, on the face of society, that by going through with certain processes of medication — in plain English, by applying to the blood certain poisons — the poisonous nature of the disease can be arrested; and if its effects do not at once disappear, it is, at least, no longer communicable. This is indeed some apology; but is it sufficient? Would a young man, on entering into matrimony, in such circumstances, with the effects of a terrible disease still, in some measure, adhering to him, be doing as he would wish to be done by? Would he not, in similar circumstances, expect the diseased individual to wait a little while?

Nothing appears to me more plain than the duty of waiting, a little time, in these circumstances, instead of proceeding headlong, as soon as a few doses of mercury have been swallowed. Or if a young man is determined not to wait at all, but rush at once, into hymeneal bands, he ought at least to reveal the circumstances in which he has placed himself. To do less, as I think, would be to forfeit every ordinary claim to common truth and honesty; and to lay himself open to all the guilt which I have, in the preceding paragraphs, alluded to.

I can, indeed, conceive of a case, in which an inoffensive young man may fall into sin and consequent suffering, and yet become truly penitent afterwards. Such a young man will act the part of the penitent if he has sense enough to know what that part is. In any event, he knows what it is not. He knows, very well, that it is not acting the part of a penitent to enter into married life without letting his companion know something of his own history; and if she has had no opportunity of access to it, before, of his general character.

The truth is, that honesty should be applied to this whole matter of courtship and marriage, as well as to matters of mere business. I like exceedingly the following story which, in its essential facts, may be relied on. It might, by a little transposition, become a part of our chapter on the errors of courtship.

A worthy citizen of New England's metropolis, became attached to a beautiful young lady, and without sufficient consideration offered her his hand. But there was a stain on her character, which time had not yet effaced; of which he was ignorant. In a thoughtless hour she had purloined some property from a shop, and had been detected. The crime was so well known and the offence betrayed so much of depravity that the distressed parents were about to spurn her from their home, when by the intercession of a friend, they retained her; and she ever afterwards acted the part of a true penitent. When offers of marriage were made her, she revealed the substance of these facts to her lover. This very honesty overcame him; the offer of his hand was repeated, and with new earnestness; and they became, in the sequel, a happy couple, and are now bringing up, in the nurture and admonition of the Lord, a happy family.

But I do not think we should expect such honesty and conscientiousness on the part of a young man who has had the venereal disease. It is not, in this matter, as it is with masturbation. Young men are not fully impressed with the idea — they never have been — that masturbation, in every degree, is wrong, just as truly wrong as fornication. There is a lingering belief abroad that though the illicit intercourse of the sexes, in every instance and degree, is sinful, yet such is the male constitution that occasional solitary indulgence is hardly wrong. The evil is supposed to lie, as with rum, in excess, and not in moderation. And this, as with the friends of temperance in regard to rum, leaves them at liberty to indulge a little now and then; and yet maintain a comparatively good conscience.

But with regard to illicit social indulgence, every enlightened and truly conscientious person is fully aware of its guilt. In this view, therefore, there is no apology for the sin, not even for one transgression. With this admission — and who is there that will not be ready and willing to make it — we remove, at once, all apology for the venereal disease. If social indulgence, out of wedlock, is wrong — is truly guilty — then he who contracts the venereal disease out of wedlock, is truly guilty, and ought to suffer the heaven-appointed penalty.

It is to be feared, after all, that the great majority of those who communicate this disease, in any of its forms, to their wives at home, neither are now, nor have ever been, truly conscientious men. It is, at all events, to be presumed that in exposing the virtuous and the innocent, they are not conscientious; especially in exposing them to a species of suffering that besides the feeling of self-abhorrence it induces, is, at best, tedious and sometimes absolutely intolerable.

CHAPTER XIII.

DIRECTIONS TO PARENTS AND GUARDIANS.

The general truth, that he who would be most useful, most honorable, most healthful and most happy, in life, must enter, at a suitable age, into marriage, has been sufficiently asserted, and reiterated. Indeed it seems so obvious a truth that one is almost ready to apologize for asserting it at all.

But he who shall enter into matrimonial life, as a man of honor and principle, may reasonably expect to hold a station of power and influence. In fact, it cannot be otherwise. As sons, wards, clerks, apprentices, or journeymen, he will, almost inevitably have around him, at all times a greater or smaller number of young men. He may, as a teacher, or in some other situation of responsibility, have around him and dependent on him, not a few, merely, but some scores or hundreds.

Now in his contact with young men, under any or all these circumstances, he will and must have more or less of influence. This influence he can make promote the cause of good and truth, or that of evil and falsehood — just as his heart may be inclined to the one or the other. But the power to exert an influence for good or for evil, involves responsibility. This responsibility, young men who enter matrimonial life must expect. They cannot escape it, if they would. Even if they should escape the charge of very *small* children, they cannot wholly escape that of those who are older. In some form or other, they will be apt to have the charge of young men, who are as much more difficult to shape properly, as their passions and appetites are stronger or more excitable.

In short, those for whom this book was prepared, will, as a general rule, in their turn, have the care of the young. Suppose, now, you have fairly got beyond the dangers of youth and childhood — aye, and if you please, manhood, too — so that all, or nearly all I have written, thus far, has been of no service to you, with regard to your own health; you may, perhaps, profit from what remains, in its application to those whom you love or esteem.

Suppose you are entrusted with the care of sons and daughters. The education and particular management of the daughters, you will, almost as a matter of course, leave to others, especially to your wife — only reminding her, from time to time, of the dangers, in general, which beset them, here and there; begging her to be constant, in season and out of season, in her endeavors to escape them.

For yourself, you will proceed, as soon as possible, to the great work of endeavoring to prevent that tissue of miseducation, misinformation, and misguidance to which you were yourself early subjected; and to give to your sons, and those dependent on you, from time to time, as their opening years may require, such instruction and guidance as God, in making you a father, or master, intended you should bestow — which, moreover, might have saved *you*, had it been applied properly, many a pang, as well as many a bitter tear of remorse. Or if you have clerks, apprentices, wards, or pupils in your family, whose age and circumstances and dangers require your care, you will not fail to perceive the necessity — I mean now the duty — of having an eye to their right management and instruction.

You will not, of course — at least you need not — make the somewhat frequent mistake of not adapting your instructions to their age, circumstances, and necessities. You will remember the good old-fashioned and common sense rule of " here a little and there a little, as they may be able to bear it."

I knew the father of a large family in the city of Hartford, who made it a principle to begin with his sons, in this matter, at eight years of age. On asking him if his efforts were not somewhat premature, his reply was that Satan did not think so — that through the medium of ungodly, profane, and wickedly obscene school-boys, bad seed had been sown in their hearts, already; and it was high time to attend to them. And I know of no man whose success, in this preventive department of physical education, was greater.

Nor is this the only instance I have known where similar success, by similar means, has been obtained; though I am obliged to confess that instances of the kind are by no means as numerous as I could wish they were. But there are a few here and there, widely scattered.

A father who would accomplish the greatest amount of good in his power, by this preventive course of instruction, should labor in season and out of season, to secure the full confidence of his sons, clerks, wards, or apprentices, so that in all their trials, difficulties, temptations, or failures, they may not shrink from the duty of coming to them at once, and unbosoming themselves, and asking for that counsel or aid which the circumstances of the case demand.

One of the fathers I have alluded to, told me that he gained the point which seems to me so desirable — that of making his sons feel full confidence in him, and take him for their most intimate friend — in such perfection, that whenever their amativeness or alimentiveness became unduly and undesirably active, they did not hesitate for a moment, to come to him and ask him to aid them in restoring their systems to such a condition that the higher law of the mind could regain and hold its wonted supremacy. How much evil may have been prevented, in this way, eternity only can make fully known.

You will ask, perhaps, and very naturally, what are some of the steps to be taken in this matter. In other words, suppose a boy eight years of age is to be conversed with; how should we begin?

I will present you, in as brief space as possible, with the essentials of a course which has been taken with boys of this age; and even with those who are younger. In your own family you may not be able to follow it implicitly; and yet it will afford you many hints. Nor does it require, as you may at first be led to suppose, large measures of physiological knowledge. A little acquaintance with the human system, — the house we live in, — with a large amount of good sense, and a hearty desire to do good, are all the qualifications for the work which are indispensably necessary.

Observe, however, that though the narrative part is professedly put into the mouth of a father, it is not intended to affirm that I have repeated every word of the conversation just as it took place; but only the substance of it to the best of my present recollection and ability.

"An inquisitive little boy, say six or seven years of age, being in the room with me one day, just after dinner, I asked him whether he had eaten anything that day. O yes! was his reply; I have eaten breakfast and dinner. And where is your dinner now? I said. He hesitated, but at length replied: I suppose it has gone down into my legs and feet, and up into my arms and head to make them grow.

"I took occasion to present him with a new and better edition of his physiology of digestion; for though he had done pretty well for a boy of his age, yet he was obviously and manifestly a little behind the times. I told him, that the food he had eaten had indeed gone into his legs, and arms, and all parts of his system, to make them grow; but not till it had been worked up, in his stomach and intestines and lungs, into blood.

"This was, perhaps, the first time he had ever thought of machinery in his "house;" and, even now, he had not thought of an architect. So I told him further that only a part of what he had eaten had been made into blood. You swallowed, I observed to him, some of the skins and seeds of your apple. Now, when you swallow such things as these they cannot be made up into blood. You sometimes, also, eat more than the digestive machinery can work up. In these cases, and to prevent these substances from accumulating and giving us trouble, they are carried out of the body.

"To facilitate the process of conducting off the waste parts of our food, and substances which cannot be dissolved at all, the great Creator has provided a long crooked channel or pipe in our bodies, called the intestinal canal. The stomach is a part of it, only it is, as it were, swelled out, or enlarged, at the place where your food and drink are first received. The intestinal canal, in a grown person, is almost two rods long. Now all the waste food and undissolved substances we take into our stomachs, are carried out of the body through this pipe.

"At a second conversation, in continuation of the subject, I spoke of drinks, and of the necessity of a conduit, or sluice, to carry off the waste liquids out of the system; and briefly described it. One prominent object was to lead his mind, by the observance of design, up to a designer, or Creator; to refer him to laws; and to extend the domain of conscience.

"It was reserved to another conversation to speak of the penalties which God, in his providence, has annexed to our frequent violations of his laws, with respect to the conduits, or sluices, of the human system; such as neglecting to masticate our food, eating between meals, using too much sugar, and other saccharine substances, etc. I also told him something about flatulence, acidity, heart-burn, costiveness, diarrhœa, etc., as the penalties of violated law.

"In this, and subsequent conversations, I also said something of what physiologists call defecation, and of the necessity or duty of promptly attending to Nature's call at the outlets of these great internal channels of the body; and spoke of the penalties which God has annexed to our neglect of attention to these calls or indications.

"I soon found that I had succeeded in impressing on his mind, the idea of law, in connection with the organs of digestion: so that when he thought of any of the parts of the body that had the remotest connection with this function, he thought of God, the Creator. I was, of course, encouraged, and led to proceed to the execution of my plan. I was anxious to enthrone the Deity, so to speak, in this his rightful province and to associate him with all his numerous possessions therein.

"Months passed away; nay, I might almost say years, before I went so far as to speak to him of any other uses of the great outlets of the body, in man or woman, other than those I have already mentioned. This was as it should have been. There is no need of haste. We must sometimes think of a sentiment of the poet, Milton; that on occasions, "they best serve God, who wait.

"When he became eight or nine years of age, and began to be exposed to erroneous influences from without,— in the various forms of conversation, books, pictures, wanton songs, etc., — I did not hesitate to explain to him in plain, but correct language, other laws of the human system, and other penalties. In due time, by little and little, I pointed out to him the dangers which would follow those violations of law to which he would, from time to time, be tempted by his associates, or by his own depraved appetites and passions; and, as I fondly hoped, arrayed his judgment and conscience against them.

"By proceeding with him thus cautiously, step by step, I hoped to prevent a part, at least, of those errors to which most boys are subjected in their early education, and by early bad associates; and, at the same time, avoid awakening on the other hand those prurient feelings, and that prurient curiosity, which are so common in society, and against which it is so desirable to guard. I did not, it is true, entirely avoid the latter danger; but the conscience, as I trust, had obtained such a hold that the body was, for the most part, kept under; and a measure, at least, of that purity preserved which, during early life, is so often prostrated, if not sacrificed."

Boys, trained in this way, are easily prepared, perhaps by the age of ten or twelve, for such instruction about the great end and designs of marriage as I have given in the early chapters of this book; and, at a little later age, for all those subsequent instructions which are little, if any, less needful. And if we do not gain, by our efforts, all we could desire, we may, at the least, hope to gain something.

It will, doubtless, sometimes happen that, after you have done your best, — after you have fortified your son's purity of character as well as you know how, — the old Adam will still be stronger than the young Melancthon; at least, temporarily. Your son or pupil may come to you, and complain of a lecherous tendency manifested, as it may be, both in his sleeping and waking hours; and he may, very properly, inquire of you what he can do to avert or avoid it.

In such an exigency, you ask him about his diet and drink, and his clothing by night and by day, — about his books, his associates generally, but especially his female society. You may possibly ascertain that his diet is too stimulating; that his drink is taken hot; that he sleeps on feathers or under thick comfortables; that he has bad associates, male or female; or that his books are of a licentious character. By the latter, however, I do not mean books of the grossest sort, for these, it is greatly and fondly to be hoped, he would not incline to; but such books as some of those which may be found in nearly all of our bookstores and libraries, but which do not always deserve a place so conspicuous.

It will be exceedingly gratifying to a father, and will more than repay him all the trouble it costs, to find his sons, wards, pupils, clerks, and apprentices thus making him a confidant, and consulting him in matters in regard to which most of the young are accustomed to consult, in preference, the emissaries of the Prince of Darkness. But the time may yet come when many fathers shall be so wise as to attain to this signal honor.

And yet after having done all in our power,—perhaps with entire success,—a new dependent may come under our care, in the form of an apprentice or clerk, whose habits were ruined at his arrival. And if we succeed in gaining his confidence it is, perhaps, only to know that he has been abused by quacks, or is abusing himself by his fears.

I have spoken elsewhere of land-sharks. Our young apprentice or clerk has fallen, it may be, into a shark's mouth; and the usual consequences have followed. I need not point out to you the road to be pursued in such cases as regards medical treatment, because I have said all I intended to say, on this subject, in Chapter V. Of his treatment with regard to health generally, — and this, after all, is substantially nearly the *whole medical treatment*, — I shall have occasion to say something presently.

One of the most frequent troubles you will hear of, — I mean during, or in connection with, these confidential disclosures, — will be the very common, and very ancient one, of nocturnal emissions. But having treated of these at considerable length elsewhere, and said that it is not the emissions, themselves, to which we must direct our attention, but the means of restoring bodily health and vigor, I shall proceed immediately to the particular consideration of that subject.

Of course it is taken for granted here, that the prominent or first cause of all the trouble complained of is forever laid aside; for, otherwise, nothing effectual is done, or can be. The most important part of repentance is reformation, — in these matters, as well as in morals.

I have remarked in Chapter VII, that the consumptive and nervous are much more inclined to sexual indulgence than other people. The truth is, that consumptive and nervous people are very much given up to the pursuit of indulgences of every sort. Who will show us any good? is, practically, their continual cry. Something they demand perpetually, to satisfy a nervous craving. They are hungry, and must eat often, or, at least, just taste a little. They are thirsty, and must drink. Their stomachs feel badly, and they must take something — I mean of the medicinal kind. If alcohol or tobacco happen to be unfashionable or interdicted, and they are not in the region of ale, wine, cider, beer, tea or coffee, a little lemonade or soda water may answer the purpose. Or, in infancy and childhood, confectionery, nuts, and fruits may, for the most part, satisfy their craving.

Then there are mental cravings, which appear to have the same end in view, namely, to tickle the nerves, and thus answer the general cry or demand which I have mentioned in the last paragraph. And, in answer to this demand of the mental stomach, the land swarms with newspapers and picture books and yellow covered literature, — as did Egypt, of old, with flies and locusts.

Well do I remember a poor consumptive man of fifty years ago, — for he was the only consumptive person I knew in those days of consumptive scarcity, — who was the very personification of the characteristics of which I am speaking. Greatly vicious, indeed, I do not say that he was, for he had not energy enough to be so; but there was the latent propensity, and the matter seemed to be well understood all over the neighborhood.

But this young man's thirst for sensuous indulgence extended to almost every thing. He was excessively fond of hot drink of every sort; and the more stimulating it was, the better it pleased him. He was equally fond of hot and greasy food, hot rooms, and hot beds.* And his indulgent friends did

* Had he lived half a century later, he would have relished

not scruple to furnish him, now and then, with a little hot toddy, or some other medicinal mixture, such as they supposed the delicacy of his constitution and his particular complaint demanded.

In truth, the common sense of the community, even at that time, — rude and uncultivated as that common sense itself was, — seems to have been nearly in unison with the decisions of science at the present hour. It was said to me, repeatedly, by my good mother (who feared the approach of pulmonary consumption), whenever I was about to indulge myself with hot biscuit and butter, hot short cake, dough-nuts, chicken-pie, mince-pie, high-seasoned food, or hot tea and coffee: "Now, my child, remember consumptive people are always fond of hot things." But "consumptive people," in my narrow vocabulary, meant Mr. Harmon, our neighbor; and the thought that I might, perchance, have consumption, and look as emaciated, and cough as dreadfully as he, kept my hands away from hot food and drink to an extent that even now, in the recollection, gives me much satisfaction.

The young man who has fallen into the habit of self-pollution will, almost of a certainty be found greatly attached to hot and exciting food and drink. He will not be apt to relish plain water, or good bread and fruits, — I mean as a means of meeting and satisfying the natural demands of the system. He

most keenly air-tight stoves. They are better fitted for su persons as he than for anybody else, though better adapted in the same degree, to destroy them.

will, indeed, use water to cool himself when hot, and to dilute his other and more stimulating beverages; and fruits, as indulgences, especially at unseasonable hours; but he would almost as soon perish as follow out such a prescription as the nature of the case would require.

Hence it is, in part, that young men fall into those merciless hands of which I have already spoken. They are far more willing to pursue the path of their natural inclinations, and then, by way of atonement, fall into a shark's mouth, than to exercise a little self-denial for a few weeks or months, and prevent such a painful necessity.

But the wise father, who has so far gained the confidence of his dependent as to make him desirous of conversation on the subject, must seize his opportunity to do what the nature of the case requires. He must must endeavor to make him understand the indispensable necessity of his using no other drink but plain water, and no other food than the plainest and most digestible viands.

Among these, good plain bread, — usually of unbolted meal, — of suitable age, with ripe fruits, cooked or otherwise, as may be most convenient, are, in general, to be preferred. To these, however, may be added some of the more digestible of the garden and field vegetables and roots, such as beans, peas, turnips, parsnips, carrots, and squashes; and, in moderation, beets and potatoes. Some very few of the foreign farinaceous substances and fruits are also admissible, — such as rice, sweet potatoes, arrow root, sago, tapioca, olives, dates, etc.

Such of the garden and field vegetables as are improved by cookery — and most of them undoubtedly are — should be prepared in a plain and simple manner; and be partaken of in the form of two or three, but never more than three meals a day. I have elsewhere alluded to some of the mischiefs resulting from the use of improper food, and bad cookery; it remains, only, that I should say, positively, what things are most useful.

The last meal of the day should be taken at least four or five hours before retiring to rest, and perhaps six would be preferable. In the latter case, however, but two meals should be allowed — one at nine or ten of the forenoon, and the other at four in the afternoon. The fewer kinds of food taken at the same meal, the better; but there should be considerable variety at different meals.

Although I am friendly to cookery — despite of the new-fangled doctrines of Dr. Schlemmer and his school — yet I am opposed, most decidedly, to all complication and abuse of this art. If our cookery cannot be simple, it were better to have none at all. Men may subsist, tolerably well, without the application of any culinary processes to their food, at least if early trained to it. And even in other circumstances, and especially for that class of invalids for whom I am now writing, I should greatly prefer no cookery at all to that eternal round of mixed dishes — pies, cakes, puddings, preserves, soups, sauces, etc., which involves, as in France, six hundred and eighty-five ways of using, as a seasoning, the egg.

Cooking is legitimate, even for invalids, when without rendering the food any less agreeable to the taste it increases its nutritious properties, or renders it more digestible. Thus the cooked potatoe is at once more nutritious and more digestible, without being less palatable, when cooked properly, than when eaten raw. But when in addition to simple cookery — roasting, baking, boiling, etc. — it is besmeared with condiments or deluged with gravies, it is injured. So milk, at least for the young, when recent, is good food; but when subjected to any process of cookery, especially when tortured into butter and cheese, it becomes difficult of digestion and is exceedingly unwholesome, especially for the lecherous, or the sensitive and delicate. It is indeed the best when most recent.

Nor should the patient, in the case before us, be permitted to use *dressings* of all sorts with his food. It were far better for him, as a general rule, that all seasonings were excluded, except perhaps, a little salt. And even this last, when it has been applied to food in the way of preserving it, is objectionable. If used at all, it should be in very small quantity, — sprinkled on our food after it is prepared and laid on our plates. In any other manner, and in any but the smallest possible quantity which is necessary to satisfy the clamorous demands of a fallen stomach, it is no other than a moderate poison to every body. Dr. Rush supposed the fabled notion that Venus rose from the sea, had its origin in the well known connection between the use of salt and *venery*.

I have alluded to the use of salt in the way of preserving food, as being injurious. Now it should be known, most fully, by every father who has the care of sensuous or debilitated young men, that all appliances to preserve food from decomposition are injurious — not merely salt, but saltpetre, smoke, spices, and even concentrated **sweets. For all** these tend to harden, if not change the texture of the food to which they are applied, especially animal food; and whatever does this to food tends to render it, at the same time more or less indigestible, and, consequently, in the same proportion likely to cause irritation, and lead to sensuality.

As to animal food, in itself considered, much might be said. In any other manner, except in the form of plain fresh steak or muscle, plainly cooked, or not cooked at all, without any dressing, except it be a *little* salt sprinkled over its surface at the table, it is decidedly objectionable for the young. And even in this way, there are few who would be so much benefited by its use as they would be by submitting to the digestive action, daily, a suitable quantity of good bread and fruits.

Of the animal products, as they are called, I have already spoken, at least in part. Butter and cheese have been wholly proscribed. Milk, recently from a healthy animal, may sometimes be allowed in the way of compromise. Eggs are to be interdicted, and still more strongly hard cooked eggs.

It is not stimulus, properly so called, that young men need, in the case before us, so much as nourishment. The mass of mankind have, however, mistaken stimulus for nutriment. Flesh and fish afford nutriment, in tolerable proportion, but they also stimulate the nervous system too much. The habit of depending on this stimulation along with our food, has led most people to confound stimulation and innervation; and if an article of food is ever so nutritious, and yet does not excite or stimulate the nerves of the stomach and of the rest of the system, it is thought to be deficient in nutrient properties. It would be strange indeed if you, who read this book, should have escaped this error.

As things are, it will be the wiser course for you, in directing the diet of debilitated young men, to labor to find out, as nearly as you can, what is *right*, and require them to follow it. Neither you nor they have reason to trouble yourselves about the degree of immediate strength which food affords. Half a gill of alcoholic liquor thrown into the stomach will sometimes give more strength for half an hour or an hour than half a pound of bread or meat. Does it therefore nourish more? By no means. It does not nourish at all. It does not contain a particle of nourishment. We mistake stimulation of the nerves, or nervous excitement, for nutrition. We mistake temporary for permanent strength. So it is with many other things.

The degree of immediate strength, therefore, which a thing affords, is far enough from being the measure of its nutritive power. Flesh and fish and high seasoned and highly concentrated dishes excite the nerves of the stomach, I say, and seem to give more strength than plain viands; but do we not mistake excitement for strength? On this point, there can, I think, be little doubt; and I need not enlarge. If what I have said is not intelligible, more would not probably be so.

Most young men, in the circumstances to which these remarks refer, are in haste to get well, and are unwilling to follow the farther but surer road. Medicine, or rather quackery, holds out the promise of a better road — better at least, because shorter. But if you can convince them that the road which is a little "farther round," is the more safe one, you will gain a great victory. Plain food and water, if faith, and hope, and cheerfulness, can go along with them, will have a far better remedial effect, without any aid from medicinal agents, than an overweening regard to medicine, while the dietetics are overlooked or disregarded. I may say still more; that if the diet and other things about to be recommended, are as they should be, no medication will often be needed. I speak here of the cure of nocturnal emissions grounded on mere debility. The occupation should be such as may be adapted to the existing degree of strength and the peculiarities of taste and general character. If possible it should be such as to give a great variety of moderate muscular exercise in the open air, and in cheerful circumstances. And if it be such as combines with other qualifications the consciousness and pleasure of *imparting good*, it will be still better adapted to the wants and circumstances of the patient.

The number of hours he should spend in labor, daily, as well as the character of the labor, will require a little thought. And here let me say what I must say somewhere, that though you may not need advice from medical men, in regard to medicine, properly so called, you may derive the most important, to you, of all information in the world, by consulting them in regard to prevention. The ordinary routine of medical practice is not to be despised; but here, in the world of prevention, is a much nobler field than that of mere cure; and happy is he who is ready and willing to enter and occupy it.

In general, the patient should be so occupied as regards the number of hours he is employed, and the degree and amount of strength he may be called upon to exert, as will be likely to secure for him the greatest amount of constitutional vigor. If it is needful to avoid the extreme of idleness, on the one hand, — involving as it necessarily would, a tendency of the mind to prey upon itself — it is equally desirable to avoid the other and worse extreme, that of over exhaustion and depression. In avoiding Scylla, it is wise, always to beware of Charybdis.

You may not always be able to change, suddenly, a young man's occupation, even where that occupation is wrong. But you may, for the most part, do *something*. If a permanent change is not practicable, a temporary change may be. Avoid, above all, an occupation that confines him too many hours in bad air, in contact as it were with a modern air-tight stove; and which keeps him sitting too much. Nor is it a small thing, in itself, physiologically, to say that he should not sit much in positions which unduly heat his body or any part of it. Sitting much with the lower limbs across each other is to be avoided.

His clothing should neither be too scanty on the one hand, nor too abundant or too irritating on the other. To go, habitually, with a chilly and shrunk skin would be to cause the blood to retreat, in a measure, from the surface towards the internal organs — perhaps to overload and excite them unduly; and as one of its results, to produce the very evil which those who have long been the slaves to masturbation are wont to dread.

On the other hand, to keep the surface of the body too warm, is no less injurious, as all experience shows than to keep it too cool. Perhaps we may not be able to explain fully the process by which such a result is effected; but there is reason for believing it is by weakening what is usually called the calorific function — by which is meant, in general, the machinery for generating heat. That machinery is, in a sense, the whole human body; but particular organs, such as the lungs, skin, and brain, are supposed to have greater calorific power than others. The lungs have been usually regarded as the great fire-place of the human system; but whether or not this is so, the stronger the lungs are the better, without a doubt.

It should be well understood by the young, particularly debilitated young men, that every degree of unnecessary heat, externally applied, whether by raising the temperature of the air in our rooms, or by adding to our clothing, has an effect at the same time, and in the same proportion, to extinguish what I here call the internal fire. In other words, it takes away from the lungs, and skin, and internal organs, — and from the system generally — their power to generate heat; so that when the fire within might otherwise keep up the bodily heat at ninety-eight or one hundred degrees, and be able to spare a good deal to the surrounding atmosphere besides, without any feelings of discomfort, it seems to act as if somewhat smothered, and the person is chilly.

The power of generating our own heat — and consequently the necessity of having strong and active bodies, — especially in a climate like ours, and in our fallen condition, is of immense importance; and woe to him who reduces it in the smallest possible degree without necessity. But this reduction is made when we wear more clothing than we really need, whether by night or by day.

It should be understood that just in proportion to our power of generating heat, is our power of casting off any excess. Sir Charles Blagden, who suffered himself to be heated gradually, in an oven, to two hundred and sixty degrees — till most substances would bake in a very short time by his side — had, of course, great power of throwing off the excessive heat, both through his skin and his lungs. But he had power, in the same proportion, of generating his own heat. At least he had this power, unless he made so many experiments of this kind as to weaken it. But after all it is not a few temporary chills or heats that weaken us, so much as the *habitual* application of a temperature higher or lower than is best for us.

Hence will be seen the great importance, to the debilitated young man, of so dressing himself by day as well as so protecting himself by night, as shall, if possible, secure to him this golden mean. He should so manage himself that instead of weakening his skin, from day to day, and subjecting himself to those *ups and downs* of temperature which so many feel, in our variable climate, his skin may be constantly growing more healthy and vigorous. The skin is a kind of safety valve to the human system; nor am I sure that, if properly attended to, the boiler would ever burst.

If it is advisable to have a proper regard to our clothing by day, it is still more so — vastly more so — to have every thing as it should be by night. Not so much, it is true, because nocturnal emissions are more frequent in hot and unventilated beds than elsewhere, though this consideration should have weight; but chiefly because too much clothing, and clothing of certain kinds which might be named, is apt to increase the general and local debility on which the emissions so largely depend.

It is a fact which not a few have noticed, that sleeping on soft feathers and down is apt to induce perspiration and weakness about the loins. We all perspire freely, as a general rule, while we sleep; but why we should be particularly weakened at the loins, is not so evident. Is it that the kidneys, being relieved of a part of their labor by the increased activity of the skin, become irritable?

I would almost as soon have a son or clerk of mine who was at all amative, or who was debilitated by amative indulgences, sleep on a hatchel as on a feather bed. Indeed, I see no reason why the former should not be preferred. The sharp points could only injure the body; they could not reach the spirit. But the unnatural and unnecessary heat, by means of an influence which if obscure and indirect is nevertheless certain, will be likely to affect the soul. For myself, I so much despise feather beds, that I would never consent to use one, except as a treat to visitors who were accustomed to them. Good husk and hair mattresses and elastic wire beds have always answered my own purpose, and that of my family.

But thick comfortables, too, are objectionable. They are too hot; and besides they do not admit of a proper change of air, and electricity. Dutch blankets are preferable. I have travelled in a region where it was customary to use two feather beds — one over, and the other underneath the occupant. Comfortables above, and feather beds beneath, are little, if any better, for the cause of purity.

Most people sleep under a great deal too much clothing. The custom is ruinous to all, but especially to the feeble in infancy and youth. It makes them tender and delicate; and, in a particular manner renders them liable to take cold.

Most persons have such a quantity of clothing on their beds as enables them to get warm almost as soon as they lie down, even in the coldest weather. They are not willing to wait a reasonable time. The result often is, that they lie all night under one third or one fourth too much covering. This is exceedingly injurious.

On stopping at a public house in the western part of Massachusetts, many years ago, I was furnished with a bed without feathers. Rejoiced to find myself for once in my life, allowed to sleep on a mattress, without "quarrelling" with my landlord, and being too much fatigued to have more than one idea in my head at a time, I forgot to notice the amount of clothing. About midnight I awaked and found myself sweltering under too much clothing. I removed just one half of it, and yet slept quite warm enough. Nor did I, while I remained there — a week or more — need more clothing than I used the first night, though the weather remained about the same.

My full and deliberate conviction is that the great mass of mankind, the civilized world over, sleep under one fourth, if not one third, more clothing than they really need, even in the coldest weather. And the more we use, the more we may; and, indeed, must,— and for a very plain reason. The more we depend on external heat, the more indolent and inefficient the internal fire becomes. And then, too, the old adage, "give an inch, and take an ell," becomes applicable here. The more indulgence we grant to the naturally indolent calorific function, the more liberty it takes of sitting still and doing nothing.

One father, whom I know, takes pains to have his sons sleep cool as a preventive of evil. He goes even farther. He never allows a young man to sleep with his arms in the bed. Such a caution might be advantageous to many older persons, as well as to the young. If it is said that we could not sleep so warmly in this position, I reply, so much the better, provided you are not chilly. Such sensations as might lead us to change our position a few times, during the night, are beneficial rather than of evil tendency.

The healthy, vigorous young man has very little occasion for going to the fire in winter, or for seeking the shade or the refrigerating cup in the summer. He is not wholly insensible to the extremes of heat and cold; but then he does not greatly suffer from them. He wears, if wise, a sufficient amount of clothing during the day-time to enable him, with suitable exercise, proper food and drink, and a cheerful state of mind, to prevent being permanently chilly; but not one iota more, if he can avoid it. He seldom or never goes to the fire; and he never allows himself to sit roasting himself by the stove or fire-place, or toasting his feet.

We do not, indeed, expect the young to turn recluse, and imitate the late Cardinal Cheverus, of Boston, or the benevolent Abbé de l'Epeé, of Europe, and go without artificial heat, in their rooms all winter, — for though such denials may be borne, I have doubts of their general usefulness. Trained as most of us have been, I think such a course would, in the end, prove too exhausting for human nature to endure. But I have a right to expect that every feeble young man who assents to the force of what I have here written will deny himself more or less, daily and hourly, instead of rushing to the fire at every slight sensation of a little cold. I expect him, moreover, to remember that for every degree of unnecessary warmth, — of warmth, I mean, which a little moderate exercise, with plain food and reasonable clothing, and patient waiting, and general cheerfulness would bring him, — in which he indulges, he must pay a future penalty in comparative delicacy and feebleness of constitution; saying nothing of the tendency of sore eyes, sore throats, lung fevers, brain fevers, peripneumony, rheumatisms, etc., in the winter; diarrhœas, and dysenteries, in summer; and asthmas, scrofulas, and consumptions, at all seasons.

Nor must young people, especially the delicate and debilitated, go suddenly to the fire when very cold. This, if done, and thousands do it, is exceedingly injurious. But I have no room in this place to enlarge and to present all the physiological reasons which might be desired.

I must, however, repeat the caution I have given with regard to excess of heat during the night; because I know of no one place in which so much mischief is done to the delicate, and sensitive, and nervous, and consumptive as in their sleeping-chambers. To roast ourselves, as it were, by fires or stoves, especially in unventilated air, is bad *enough;* but then it is not usual — it is exceedingly rare — for us to be steeped in bad air, six, eight or ten consecutive hours, any where else except in our sleeping rooms. Here, however, hardly anything is more common. Thousands and tens of thousands, young and old, immure themselves to the full extent of periods of time like these, under an amount of clothing that is every month, and week, and day crippling, as fast as possible, their calorific powers; and hastening, apace, the day of their death.

It is not well for debilitated young men to retire too early; though it would undoubtedly be worse for them to retire too late. Nor should they, as a general rule, retire at all till there is a reasonable expectation of going at once to sleep. As sleep however on occasions may, otherwise, be dreamy, I have usually advised the debilitated young man to take care to be properly fatigued before going to rest. In this view I have occasionally recommended, just before retiring, a **walk of** one, two or three miles.

The more our debilitated young men are abroad in the open air, the more they confine themselves to plain, simple, and coarse food, and, in short, the better they obey all the laws of health and physiology, and the less they depend on medicine, the better. The laws of health, duly obeyed, are more efficient than all the pills, and tonics, and bitters in the known world.

Every young man, sick or well, should have a dress for the night. This enables him to hang up his day-clothes during the hours of his rest, and his night-clothes during the day, and thus gives him, at all times, fresh and well-ventilated apparel.

Much has been said of cold bathing in these cases, and, especially, shower bathing. With a little good, sound sense to be applied, cold bathing may sometimes be very serviceable; but, unless judiciously managed, it is apt to do quite as much harm as good. I have seen it tend greatly to invigorate the constitution; but I have also known it prove debilitating.

To be made beneficial, either in the particular cases we are considering, or any where else, it must be followed by what is called a reaction. In other words, it must be followed by a general warmth, if not a glow, all over the surface of the body, and by an increased buoyancy of spirits, and mental activity. No person,— unless it were a maniac,— who is made pale, cold, or, even chilly, dull, languid or melancholic by the cold-bath, will derive much benefit from it, whatever may be the other attending circumstances, or however great, in his own case, the apparent necessity of its application.

Local bathing, in the case of your debilitated son or clerk, will often do better than general bathing. Among the various forms of local bathing is the *sitz* bath. This consists simply in sitting in a tub of water usually cold, and remaining two, five or ten minutes, as may be deemed advisable on trial. The *douch*, or dash, which consists in throwing a jet of water against some part of the body, is often useful.

General bathing will often have the best effect on the debilitated, when taken on going to bed. A tub should be used; the water should be tepid or warm — from 85 to 98 degrees. The whole body, up to the head, may be immersed in the tub from ten to twenty minutes. On leaving the bath, the body should be wiped dry as quickly as possible, and should be made warm in bed as soon as possible.

In some few cases, it will be found preferable to use cold water, for general bathing, rather than warm. But this must be taken at rising in the morning, or about the middle of the forenoon. The latter is the best time to get a reaction; but the former is the most common. But even then I would not use the shower-bath; and the tub-bath is little better. Nor would I begin by bathing the whole body at once.

My method is as follows. Remove the clothing as quickly as possible, and after washing little more than the head and hands, apply coarse towels not only to the head and hands, but to the whole body. Rub well, for several minutes. If not very robust, an assistant will be needed here; and, if ever so healthy, the good strong hand of a friend will be useful. When the friction is over, apply the clothing again as quickly as possible, and use moderate but quick exercise.

The next day I proceed a little farther. I now venture to sponge the chest, before the friction. The third day I extend the water still farther. The fourth a little farther still. Thus beginning with very nearly what Dr. Franklin would call the air-bath, I gradually convert it into a general sponge-bath.

With the aid of cautions and suggestions like these, nearly every debilitated young man may derive benefit from bathing, in some of its various forms; and oftentimes from cold bathing. But, I repeat once more, — he must take care to secure a good re-action after the cold bath, or it will be of very little service to him.

In connection with the remark above, that an assistant is sometimes useful, I have an anecdote to relate, to which I beg the closest attention; for it points to a truth of great importance.

The wife of one of our most distinguished literary men was feeble, and had long been in the daily use of the cold shower-bath. As she had no help, she came out of the bathing-room, at the close, pale and wan, and exceedingly exhausted. In these circumstances, as might have been expected, she did not secure a good reaction; and, of course, remained in the same state of health; or, if there was any alteration at all, it was for the worse.

The husband saw the difficulty, and proposed a remedy. This was to relieve her from the necessity of exhausting her strength during the friction. In a word, he proposed to assist her, and the proposal was gladly accepted.

This changed the state of things entirely. Not a month elapsed ere she was able to obtain a good reaction, in every instance; and in a year or two her general health was greatly improved.

I ought to say, however, that her husband made use of his hand, as well as of a coarse towel. He was a stout, healthy man, and seemed to have a superabundance of electricity in his general system. It was a question with him, which I cannot solve, but which I leave to your consideration, how far he electrified or magnetized her; and to what extent her recovery was owing to this influence.

If a debilitated young man attends school,—and it is by no means uncommon on account of his feebleness to send him to school for a time,—great care is necessary with regard to his health while there. In the far greater proportion of our schools, little or no attention is paid to the health of the pupils, any more than if the subject had no claims whatever on the teacher's attention, or even on the parents. If the young do not actually get sick at school, no one seems to think of any delinquency. There is a great mistake here. The young, of every age, should improve in health, while at school, with just as much certainty as in knowledge, or excellency, or good behavior.

One of the most common abuses at the school-room consists in an almost entire neglect of the laws of ventilation. I do not believe one school in ten, — I speak now more particularly of our public schools, though the remark would not be inapplicable to some of our private schools, — has pure air in it for a single hour in the day.

But exercise, too, is neglected at school. The laws of amusement seem hardly beginning to be understood. Then, again, the fixtures for heating our schoolrooms, and the situation and position of the desks and benches, are anything conceivable, rather than what they should be. The hygiene of the school-room has been, as yet, but little studied.

With regard to society, it not unfrequently happens that debilitated young persons shun mankind as much as possible, especially females. They are diffident and shamefaced, at least for the most part. I have, however, known a few of a contrary character, — bold, confident, blustering and impudent. But these last will never be likely to possess enough of ingenuousness to make a mother or a father their confidant. Their confidants, if they have any, will be those landsharks to whom I have before alluded; and you may almost as well give them up, for lost, at once.

Now it is fortunate for young men, (as I have shown in other chapters), in the first place, that they have sisters, which, as you know, is the general rule.

Secondly, it is highly important that the schools of our country, for the far greater part, are made up of males and females; and that so few of them are arranged on the *convent* system. It is scarcely less important that we have, in one form or another, in almost every neighborhood, social gatherings of some sort or other.

If any of our young men could get along and maintain their health and virtue without female society, it is most clearly none of those of whom I am now speaking. For if their natural diffidence and disinclination to female society, together, perhaps, with accidental and providential privations have been already injurious to them, why should not the same isolated condition keep them so?

In any event, let them be brought into society as much as possible. Not, of course, into night parties or night sitting; for these, especially the last, would be the worst evils that could possibly befall them; but into such afternoon family meetings of the sexes as I have repeatedly suggested and recommended. These are beneficial in every point of view; but especially to our debilitated young men.

Books are society. Great care is necessary, in these days, in selecting books for the young, especially for that class of the young to whom many of our modern publications that pass current are but mild poison.

The worst class of books that could fall into the hands of debilitated young men is, undoubtedly, a part of that very class that is professedly designed for their use. "Manhood," a French work, by Deslander, is at the head of the objectionable division of this class. It contains much valuable information for a medical man; but by grouping together so many horrid "cases," appears to me to convey an impression on the youthful mind calculated to defeat its own end. They think the dangers of masturbation exaggerated. But there are numerous books and papers that, without directly encouraging sensuality, do so indirectly. The same might be said of not a few of the books in our lighter libraries; and especially of our newspapers and magazines.

The question is often asked whether such young men as those for whom the foregoing directions are intended, ought to marry. To this inquiry the French and German physiologists, and medical men almost uniformly, reply: Yes! But the true reply might be both, yes or no, according to circumstances. I mean by this, that some young men in a state of disease from self-abuse ought to marry, and others ought not.

As long as a young man is depressed and discouraged, and his mind is turned continually to what he supposes to be the source of his woes, namely the emissions, and those are increasing in frequency, or even not diminishing, he ought not to think of marriage, except in a general or philosophic way. I make this last exception, because I have already advanced the opinion, more than once, that the young ought by all means, as a general rule, to look forward to matrimony. A state of disease, however, sometimes forbids this, so far as to think of it as very near at hand.

When, however, things take a better turn, and the young man begins to have a little courage; when it becomes obvious that he has passed quite beyond the "slough of despond," as Bunyan calls it, and has begun to gain the ascent beyond it, then he may be encouraged to marry. The hope of being able to do so, will now prove a healthful stimulus to him. It is true that he must not place the day of consummation too near; nor is it necessary. The hope of being a husband, and of enjoying the society of a wife, though many years distant, will be far better than downright discouragement and dejection. [See Appendix A.]

Why is it that our writers on this subject do not discriminate? True it is that they cannot reach the particulars of every case, were it ever so desirable; but there are often a few leading principles, that should be laid down and adhered to, like the foregoing.

There is one thing more to be mentioned that will greatly aid a young man in recovering health and vigor. It is the love of improvement. Our rules of improving the body are of little value, — I had almost said none at all to those for whom they are given, — unless there is coupled with the rest a burning desire to become wiser and better, no less than healthier. For all our efforts to obtain health, unless in order that we may be good and useful, what are they but sheer selfishness? And though selfish men may improve in health and vigor, yet they will not make half as much progress, other things and circumstances being equal, as benevolent ones.

I know not exactly how it is, — but there is something in human selfishness that not only tends to narrow and contract the feelings, but to impair the bodily health at the same time. Or if the effect is so slow as not to be readily perceptible, it is none the less certain. It is not too much to say that under the influence of benevolent feelings, when a person is not too far gone, all the organs of the body will slowly gain strength; and that this is true even of the skin and bones.

Though it forms no part of the plan of this volume to inculcate morals and religion, yet I must be permitted to say that it will add much to our influence, in endeavoring to recover a fallen young man, if we can be successful in bringing him to the practical benevolence of the Gospel, and making him a true follower of the Lord Jesus Christ. HE was evidently healthy; and a part of this, at the least, was the natural reward of his untiring practical benevolence.

CHAPTER XIV.

GENERAL DIRECTIONS TO ALL WHO ARE CONCERNED.

No man, whatever, in any age of the world, has written more pointedly against licentiousness, in nearly all its varied forms, — from sodomy to polygamy, — than Paul. From Romans to Titus, all the way, we find him inculcating the necessity of "keeping under the body," lest it should obtain the mastery over the spirit, and prove the destruction of soul and body both.

Some may think the world has grown wiser and better since the days of Paul; and, in many respects, it may be so. But young men are more sanguine in this belief than older ones. The latter are forced to the conclusion, every day they live, that there is great need of laboring, as Paul did, to keep under the body, and bring it into subjection to law, physiological, no less than moral.

John Elliot, sometimes called the Indian Apostle, more than two hundred years ago, was anxious to procure a professor of anatomy and physiology, to teach the Natick Indians the laws of their bodies, and how to keep them under. He saw most clearly the practical impossibility of making good Christians of men who knew nothing of themselves.

It is true, he failed to accomplish his object; and it is also true that there was something a little visionary in his plan. It was not anatomy and physiology that the savages needed so much as a few of the simple laws of hygiene, or health. Anatomy and physiology are necessary to certain classes and professions of men; but not to everybody. And those boards of education, who have recommended them to be taught to everybody by placing them among the elementary studies of our common schools, have acted, in the premises, without a proper understanding of the subject. It is not the structure of our bodies, — the machinery, so to call it, — that is so indispensably necessary; nor the functions, or, in other words, the play of that machinery, — but how to keep the machinery in proper condition.

I admit, indeed, that a knowledge of the structure and functions of the body — anatomy and physiology — would be of some service to every individual of every age; and so would many other sciences which could be named. But life is not long enough for everybody to learn everything. Besides, a knowledge of the laws of our bodies, such a knowledge as will enable us to take care of ourselves, may be obtained nearly as well without anatomy and physiology, as with them.

How convenient it would be for everybody to know how to make their own clothes, shoes, furniture, houses, etc., but is it practicable? Is it best? How convenient it would be for all mankind to understand the nature of disease and of medicine, so as to be their own physician? But is that practicable? is life long enough? I do not think it is. Neither do I think that life is long enough for everybody to study anatomy and physiology.

As the world and things now are, we get a smattering of these sciences, unavoidably. We cannot read books and newspapers and magazines of the day, otherwise. They are a system of instruction, so to speak, on all subjects. Through their instrumentality every one, as a general rule, obtains a *universal*, if not a *university* education. I say every one, because almost every family, except a few of the very poorest, read newspapers. Most read, or at least look over, several. Indeed, nothing is more common than for a family to take a daily paper; and not a few families receive from five to fifteen periodicals of all sorts and kinds.

Grant, indeed, that, as Bacon says, a little knowledge is a dangerous thing. Still, the little knowledge-period must be passed through. The time has been when knowledge was the property of a few. It was not deemed safe to give knowledge to the mass of the people, even religious knowledge. But republicanism is now the order of the day; to some extent it is so, under despotic governments. The decree has gone out, from the Eternal Throne, that man shall be educated; and, in governments like our own, the decree is beginning to be obeyed. The press is educating us. The press is the people's college. It is, at least, a *pioneer* college. And as I said before, it already brings almost everybody within its influence.

And among the things which have so long been secluded from the common people, as useless to them, is a knowledge of the laws which regulate their own bodies. It is not yet a quarter of a century since those who controlled the public press, even in enlightened Boston, opposed the idea which a few minds had then conceived of teaching hygiene or the laws of health, to the mass of mankind, as not only a useless scheme, but an injurious one. And when the Library of Health, a monthly journal that sought to inculcate a knowledge of the laws of health began its career, twenty years ago, there was but one physician in Boston who was quite ready to bid it God speed; nor but one man in New England quite ready to subscribe for it.

That journal, with others of kindred spirit together with a few books in the same spirit has so changed the tone of the public feeling, that there is a general demand for this sort of instruction, and everybody avows himself in its favor. Indeed we are going over to the opposite extreme — as I have already intimated — and demanding not only that every one shall understand Hygiene or the Laws of Health, but Anatomy and Physiology besides. Further still, even, some are going, and demanding that every one shall become his own physician. But after a few vibrations, backward and forward, the pendulum will probably rest midway between the two extremes.

The public demand, I say, for instruction in hygiene, is so strong, that nearly every periodical responds in one way or another. One responds by noticing some new work that professes to teach hygiene to families; another by noticing a new school book on this subject, another still by original or extracted articles on health; some of which are hardly worth reading; while here and there one is valuable. But the far greater portion of the controllers of the public press are far more ready and willing to aid in selling something that professes large powers of cure, in one department or another, rather than that which teaches the way of prevention. The truth is, that there is yet a vast deal of ignorance with regard to the kinds of knowledge which is really demanded.

But along with every deduction, drawback, and difficulty, we are making many advances. The press has raised the standard of knowledge so that nearly every individual knows something of everything; and this *smattering* of everything is fast maturing into a *general knowledge* of everything.

The knowledge of hygiene has so far advanced that most persons have attained to some of the plainer principles of the science, and taken them for granted. Thus every one, or almost every one, knows that water is best adapted to quench thirst, and that distilled and fermented drinks are of doubtful tendency. That plain, simple, unstimulating food is better for health than rich, high-seasoned or complicated dishes. That tobacco, opium, and all other drugs and medicines, are more or less hurtful to everybody in health; that we should breathe pure air freely; that we should use abundant exercise; and that we should neither go habitually chilly, or too much heated, by night or by day.

These and many more of the simple laws of hygiene, are now, I say, common property. Everybody understands them. I have addressed this book to young men with the presumption that they understand them. They cannot have lived in the world during the last fifteen, or twenty, or twenty-five years, without understanding them.

Except, therefore, in the single chapter which precedes this, I have said very little about the laws of hygiene — above all, those of physiology. The latter — I repeat — I deemed hardly necessary; the former I have taken for granted, were pretty well understood. Besides, had I stopped to teach the laws — or even to point to them — as I passed along, it would have swelled my book to a much greater size than I had intended.

Perhaps too, some would, in that case, have called it a *learned* book; when my object was simply to make it plain and intelligible. Those who have no more than that mere smattering of hygiene which hardly any body can help possessing, will almost certainly understand me; and those who are more learned, of *course*, can.

In short, I think no one who reads the work thoroughly will fail to perceive that he cannot but be a very great gainer by devoting a little time to the study of himself — at least so far as the plain laws of health are concerned. Lectures, such as he may have opportunity to attend, will greatly assist him; but having been stirred up by lectures, and by the little that has been well said to him here or elsewhere, he will doubtless feel his need of farther information. That information, fortunately, can now be had, in forms which are intelligible. The only great difficulty will be in making a selection.

Among the more reliable forms of instruction, which is afforded to the young at the present day, one which should be hailed with great joy by every friend of truth and humanity, is found in the increasing tendency of medical men to address the public on subjects for which they are better prepared, other things being equal, than any other class of citizens. This fountain of correct information, it is fondly hoped will ere long be opened more widely and more extensively than it ever yet has been. [See Appendix B.]

One of the *savans* of Massachusetts — himself a medical man by education — has been heard to say, that such lectures as those I have just alluded to, and from men whom we know and in whom we are accustomed to confide, are needful every week in every school district of our wide-spread country.

This blessing however will be likely to be somewhat limited in its application, by that vulgar, not to say wicked prejudice, which so extensively prevails against every form of hygienic instruction which could be named, even that which is least exceptionable; but especially against those forms which are particularly intended for the young. The writer of this work has suffered in the estimation of his best friends, in this very way; nor has he suffered alone. He could name in this connection half a score of others.

It is not long since I received from a physician of the highest standing in one of the United States, a most interesting letter, which, in some of its aspects, develops facts concerning the public prejudice of which I am speaking, which seem a little unpropitious to the cause of human advancement, but are yet in perfect keeping with the sentiments of the preceding paragraphs. Although the letter was never intended for the public eye, yet to confirm the heavy charges I have made against the ignorance and apathy of those who have the care of the young, I venture on the following extract. The reader will perceive some of the difficulties under which preventive men labor.

"I feel a good deal as you express yourself, as if I would like to be an Apostle of Health to the great mass of humanity, and it is difficult for me now to restrain myself within the narrow enclosure of those private pursuits which the support of a family imperatively demands. It is a most inviting field of labor, but requires a fortune to work it.

"I first became warmly interested in this subject about fifteen years ago, when I was unexpectedly appointed by the Common Council, to the office of ———, an office which I held only ten months, but which excited a taste for sanitary study which time and observation of the general ignorance of the subject has only rendered more intense. I believe, however, I have been pecuniarily a great loser by that "little brief authority;" for my general reputation, thereby attained, as a devotee to matters of public interest, has interfered not a little with my reputation as a practitioner, by which craft I live.

" On this account I have of late years, rather avoided much public exposition of my name in connection with the subject; and must continue to hide my light, feeble as it is, under the bushel, unless I can manage to connect with the preaching of the subject, the receipt of a good salary."

Strange, indeed, that it should be so; but so it is. Everywhere we hear the old adage that " an ounce of prevention is worth a pound of cure;" and yet the man who devotes himself to preventing disease must suffer in his reputation and purse; while he who devotes himself to the work of cure may receive, and does receive, both a good salary and a good reputation.

But let us not by any means despair. There is — there must be — a better day coming. Truth is mighty, and must ultimately prevail. Prevention must yet have its day, or all else, even truth itself, is sheer mockery. It cannot but be seen and realized, that, in the language of a motto to one of our medical and surgical journals. "The best part of the medical art, is the art of avoiding (i. e. preventing) pain."

The young shall yet be duly cared for, and their just rights accorded to them. It is quite too much to deal out to them in every form from day to day empty compliment, concerning their importance and influence, especially when we wish to gain, at least in prospect, more or less of political or other local capital. It is time that our professed regard for the young should *mean* something. It is time to feed them with that which is bread, and will endure. If they are to bear, in their turn, the public burdens, let them be duly prepared for it; and let their bodies be attended to, no less than their minds. The value of the sound mind can never be duly appreciated, except when lodged in the sound body; nor can the moral man be greatly advanced while the physical man is so sadly neglected.

APPENDIX A.

On the subject of keeping the thoughts away from forbidden objects, as a means of restoration, the following paragraphs, derived from Dr. Carpenter's Physiology, page 465, will be found worthy of careful consideration; and though primarily addressed to medical students, and being chiefly on fornication, are applicable to all young men and to all the forms of impurity: —

"The sexual secretions are strongly influenced by the condition of the mind. When it is frequently and strongly directed towards objects of passion, these secretions are increased in amount to a degree which may cause them to be a very injurious drain on the powers of the system. On the other hand, the active employment of the mental powers on other objects has a tendency to render them less active; or even to check altogether the processes by which they are elaborated.

"This is a simple physiological fact, but of high moral application. The author would say to those of his younger readers who urge the wants of nature as an excuse for the illicit gratification of the sexual passions; try the effects of a close application to some of those ennobling pursuits to which your profession introduces you, in combination with vigorous bodily exercise, before you assert that the appetite is unrestrainable and act upon that assertion. Nothing tends so much to increase the desire as the continual direction of the mind towards the objects of its gratification. The following observations, which the author believes to be strictly correct, are extracted from a valuable little work addressed to young men. They are directed to those who maintain that the married state being natural to man, illicit intercourse is necessary for those who are prevented by circumstances from otherwise gratifying the sexual passion.

"When the appetite is naturally indulged, that is, in marriage, the necessary energy is supplied by the nervous stimulus of its natural accompaniment of love, which prevents the injury which would otherwise arise from the increased expenditure of animal power. And, in like manner, the function being in itself grateful, this personal attachment performs the further necessary office of preventing immoderate indulgence, by dividing the attention through the numerous other sources of sympathy and enjoyment which it simultaneously opens to the mind. But when the appetite is irregularly indulged, that is, in fornication, for want of a healthful vigor of true love, its energies become exhausted; and for the want of numerous other sympathetic sources of enjoyment in true love, or similar thoughts, common pursuits, and above all, in common holy hopes, the more gross animal gratification of lust is resorted to with unnatural frequency, and thus its powers become still further exhausted, and therefore still more unsatisfying, while at the same time a habit is thus created, and these jointly cause an increased craving; and the still greater deficiency in the satisfaction experienced in its indulgence further, continually, ever in a circle, increases — the habit, demand, indulgence, consequent exhaustion, diminished satisfaction, and again demand — till the mind and body alike become disorganized."

To the foregoing remarks and quotation, Dr. Carpenter also appends the following statement, which is at least as applicable to the United States as to Great Britain; and involves considerations which furnished one strong argument for the publication of the foregoing work.

"The author regrets to be obliged further to remark, that some recent works which have issued from the medical press, contain much that is calculated to excite, rather than to repress, the propensity; and that the advice sometimes given by practitioners to their patients, is immoral as well as unscientific."

APPENDIX B.

In confirmation of the truth of my remarks, as well as in proof of the usefulness of the instruction of this volume to young men under fifteen years of age, it may not be amiss to observe that but the other day the author had a letter from a young man in one of our best colleges, on the subject of giving a lecture or two for the benefit of his associates in that institution, who may not improbably be greatly indebted for his present excellency and purity of his character, to a lecture which he heard from me, at the age of fourteen, in one of the villages of southern Massachusetts. Though my advertisements excluded him, his aged, and as I trust, now sainted father, came to me and requested, as a special favor, to be permitted to bring 'this son.' He said he was not aware of any particular necessity in the case; but he was a full believer in the great doctrine of *prevention*. And it is my present strong conclusion that imperfect as the lecture may have been, both the father and the son *had their reward*.

But anecdotes and statements, of the same general character, might be multiplied to almost any extent, in a world where sin has entered, and in a soil in which it is wont to luxuriate.

Medicine & Society In America

An Arno Press/New York Times Collection

Alcott, William A. **The Physiology of Marriage.** 1866. New Introduction by Charles E. Rosenberg.

Beard, George M. **American Nervousness: Its Causes and Consequences.** 1881. New Introduction by Charles E. Rosenberg.

Beard, George M. **Sexual Neurasthenia.** 5th edition. 1898.

Beecher, Catharine E. **Letters to the People on Health and Happiness.** 1855.

Blackwell, Elizabeth. **Essays in Medical Sociology.** 1902. Two volumes in one.

Blanton, Wyndham B. **Medicine in Virginia in the Seventeenth Century.** 1930.

Bowditch, Henry I. **Public Hygiene in America.** 1877.

Bowditch, N[athaniel] I. **A History of the Massachusetts General Hospital: To August 5, 1851.** 2nd edition. 1872.

Brill, A. A. **Psychanalysis: Its Theories and Practical Application.** 1913.

Cabot, Richard C. **Social Work: Essays on the Meeting-Ground of Doctor and Social Worker.** 1919.

Cathell, D. W. **The Physician Himself and What He Should Add to His Scientific Acquirements.** 2nd edition. 1882. New Introduction by Charles E. Rosenberg.

The Cholera Bulletin. Conducted by an Association of Physicians. Vol. I: Nos. 1–24. 1832. All published. New Introduction by Charles E. Rosenberg.

Clarke, Edward H. **Sex in Education; or, A Fair Chance for the Girls.** 1873.

Committee on the Costs of Medical Care. **Medical Care for the American People:** The Final Report of The Committee on the Costs of Medical Care, No. 28. [1932].

Currie, William. **An Historical Account of the Climates and Diseases of the United States of America.** 1792.

Davenport, Charles Benedict. **Heredity in Relation to Eugenics.** 1911. New Introduction by Charles E. Rosenberg.

Davis, Michael M. **Paying Your Sickness Bills.** 1931.

Disease and Society in Provincial Massachusetts: Collected Accounts, 1736–1939. 1972.

Earle, Pliny. **The Curability of Insanity: A Series of Studies.** 1887.

Falk, I. S., C. Rufus Rorem, and Martha D. Ring. **The Costs of Medical Care:** A Summary of Investigations on The Economic Aspects of the Prevention and Care of Illness, No. 27. 1933.

Faust, Bernhard C. **Catechism of Health:** For the Use of Schools, and for Domestic Instruction. 1794.

Flexner, Abraham. **Medical Education in the United States and Canada:** A Report to The Carnegie Foundation for the Advancement of Teaching, Bulletin Number Four. 1910.

Gross, Samuel D. **Autobiography of Samuel D. Gross, M.D.,** with Sketches of His Contemporaries. Two volumes. 1887.

Hooker, Worthington. **Physician and Patient;** or, A Practical View of the Mutual Duties, Relations and Interests of the Medical Profession and the Community. 1849.

Howe, S. G. **On the Causes of Idiocy.** 1858.

Jackson, James. **A Memoir of James Jackson, Jr., M.D.** 1835.

Jennings, Samuel K. **The Married Lady's Companion, or Poor Man's Friend.** 2nd edition. 1808.

The Maternal Physician; a Treatise on the Nurture and Management of Infants, from the Birth until Two Years Old. 2nd edition. 1818. New Introduction by Charles E. Rosenberg.

Mathews, Joseph McDowell. **How to Succeed in the Practice of Medicine.** 1905.

McCready, Benjamin W. **On the Influences of Trades, Professions, and Occupations in the United States, in the Production of Disease.** 1943.

Mitchell, S. Weir. **Doctor and Patient.** 1888.

Nichols, T[homas] L. **Esoteric Anthropology: The Mysteries of Man.** [1853].

Origins of Public Health in America: Selected Essays, 1820–1855. 1972.

Osler, Sir William. **The Evolution of Modern Medicine.** 1922.

The Physician and Child-Rearing: Two Guides, 1809–1894. 1972.

Rosen, George. **The Specialization of Medicine:** with Particular Reference to Ophthalmology. 1944.

Royce, Samuel. **Deterioration and Race Education.** 1878.

Rush, Benjamin. **Medical Inquiries and Observations.** Four volumes in two. 4th edition. 1815.

Shattuck, Lemuel, Nathaniel P. Banks, Jr., and Jehiel Abbott. **Report of a General Plan for the Promotion of Public and Personal Health.** Massachusetts Sanitary Commission. 1850.

Smith, Stephen. **Doctor in Medicine** and Other Papers on Professional Subjects. 1872.

Still, Andrew T. **Autobiography of Andrew T. Still,** with a History of the Discovery and Development of the Science of Osteopathy. 1897.

Storer, Horatio Robinson. **The Causation, Course, and Treatment of Reflex Insanity in Women.** 1871.

Sydenstricker, Edgar. **Health and Environment.** 1933.

Thomson, Samuel. **A Narrative, of the Life and Medical Discoveries of Samuel Thomson.** 1822.

Ticknor, Caleb. **The Philosophy of Living;** or, The Way to Enjoy Life and Its Comforts. 1836.

U.S. Sanitary Commission. **The Sanitary Commission of the United States Army:** A Succinct Narrative of Its Works and Purposes. 1864.

White, William A. **The Principles of Mental Hygiene.** 1917.